Integrated Care for Complex Patients

Steven A. Frankel • James A. Bourgeois

Editors

Integrated Care for Complex Patients

A Narrative Medicine Approach

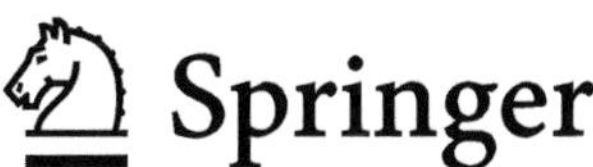 Springer

Editors
Steven A.Frankel
Department of Psychiatry
University of California
School of Medicine
San Francisco, CA, USA

James A. Bourgeois
Department of Psychiatry
Baylor Scott & White Health
Central Texas Division
Temple, TX, USA

Department of Psychiatry
Texas A and M University Health Sciences
Center, College of Medicine
Temple, TX, USA

Department of Psychiatry
University of California San Francisco
School of Medicine
San Francisco, CA, USA

ISBN 978-3-319-61212-6   ISBN 978-3-319-61214-0   (eBook)
https://doi.org/10.1007/978-3-319-61214-0

Library of Congress Control Number: 2017959589

This Springer imprint is published by the registered company Springer International Publishing AG part of Springer Nature.
The registered company address is: Gewerbestrasse 11, 6330 Cham, Switzerland

We dedicate this book to Roger Kathol, MD. Roger is truly the father of "clinical complexity." It is with his inspiration that we plan to continue to reinforce and build upon the platform he has so dedicatedly established. There is little in medicine that is more logical, more inherent, than "complexity." Systemic medicine and psychiatry combined make up only part of that picture. As Roger has shown us, the social and care delivery dimensions must be added to approach a true picture of the patient, and his or her clinical needs and circumstances. The VB IM-CAG, so much of which is Roger's creation, is a seminal blueprint for the continued development of what we hope will eventually become a "complexity specialization" within medicine.

Roger, you are not just far-seeing about medical matters, but you have laid a groundwork for the clinical practice of medicine that is both precise and at the same time humanistic. With this book we acknowledge you and celebrate your work.

Foreword

Harris Fishbon Distinguished Professor in Clinical Translational Research and Aging, Division of Geriatrics, Department of Medicine, University of California San Francisco

Health-care systems and clinicians increasingly recognize that a relatively small number of persons account for a significant amount of medical cost and utilization, with 10% of patients accounting for almost two-thirds of total health-care costs [1]. While these individuals often have multiple chronic systemic conditions and functional limitations, a major subset of these persons also has comorbid psychiatric illness and chaotic social situations. For clinicians, these individuals are "complex." Systemic medical and psychiatric illnesses, demographics, experiences with society, and the health-care system; and social capital[1] all contribute to their health status and to their illnesses. These contributing factors are interdependent and are not easily disentangled.

This population with complex care needs presents particular challenges to clinicians. As highlighted by Frankel and Bourgeois [2], their complexity can have several dimensions: diagnostic complexity, operational complexity, and management complexity. Diagnostic dilemmas arise when patients already have multiple co-occurring conditions and high symptom burden. Teasing out what symptoms represent a new condition versus a medication or ongoing illness effect can be difficult in a busy practice. Operational complexity arises when a patient with metastatic cancer also has chronic delirium, depressive disorder, and diabetes mellitus. Treatment of one condition can negatively interfere with treatments for others, and no one clinician can optimally care for a complex patient without conferring with others. Aggressive pharmacologic management of diabetes mellitus, when a person is marginally housed or treatment of heart failure without concomitant attention to comorbid psychiatric illness and nutritional support likely will fall short. Finally, management complexity is often seen in the context of comorbid personality disor-

---

[1] The networks of relationships among people who live and work in a particular society, enabling that society to function effectively.

ders impacting compliance or substance misuse. Regardless of the type of complexity, a traditional medical or biological approach to providing care to persons with complex needs offers insufficient support.

Care of persons with complex needs requires a comprehensive understanding of the wide array of factors contributing to poor wellbeing and a well-equipped interprofessional team to prioritize and address concerns. This team has to be as comfortable navigating hoarding disorder as they do navigating hypertension treatment.

For the past four decades, a variety of care delivery approaches to support persons with complex care needs have been developed and tested. Those that have shown the most benefit have included (1) comprehensive assessment of patients' needs, (2) tailored person-centered care planning based on the individual assessment, (3) support of patients in overcoming barriers to accessing needed services, (4) open and regular communication among treatment team members, (5) comprehensive care coordination, and (6) ongoing monitoring of care and care outcomes. As a geriatrician, palliative care physician, and medical director of our health system's complex care program, I have had the privilege of caring for many persons with multiple chronic serious illnesses and complex care needs. These persons have done best when assessed in the context of a biopsychosocial and spiritual framework and supported by a dedicated and well-trained team.

Until recently, however, most primary care medical practices have not been able to access many of these services. Fee-for-service reimbursement did not facilitate interprofessional care or care that is time consuming. With the advent of new payment models and the patient-centered medical home, population health-focused complex illness care programs have begun to emerge that seek to better assist patients with complex care needs. Alternative advanced payment models are designed to hold medical practices accountable for patient quality of care and cost across settings of care. Patient-centered medical homes, which evolved out of pediatrics, involve patients, caregivers, and multiple care disciplines as the care team. These care delivery models have finally provided the impetus to proactively identify those with complex care needs and to integrate effective complex care into the fabric of health care.

While it is encouraging that health systems and providers are reaching out to those most in need of holistic care, many clinicians are still poorly prepared to care for these patients. In a 2004 survey of US physicians, the majority felt inadequately prepared to care for chronically ill patients or to engage in interdisciplinary teamwork with allied health providers [3]. Even several years later, primary care clinicians express frustration about the fragmentation of care available to those with chronic complex illnesses [4]. *Integrated Care for Complex Patients: A Narrative Medicine Approach* seeks to fill these gaps and address these frustrations by providing multidimensional perspectives on complex care and strategies to manage them. It breaks down the various dimensions of complexity and highlights pragmatic approaches to manage these domains of need. In addition to explicating the many aspects of complex care, Frankel and Bourgeois provide numerous case studies that bring home important issues in the care of patients with complex care needs.

Integrated Care for Complex Patients: A Narrative Medicine Approach provides refreshing pragmatic, real-world perspectives to an increasingly important aspect of clinical care today.

Christine Ritchie, MD, MSPH, FACP, FAAHPM

References

1. Weiss KB. Managing complexity in chronic care: an overview of the VA state-of-the-art (SOTA) conference. J Gen Intern Med. 2007;22 Suppl 3:374–8.
2. Frankel SA, Bourgeois JA, Xiong G, et al. The medical-psychiatric coordinating physician-led model: team-based treatment for complex patients Psychosomatics. 2014;55(4):333–342.
3. Darer JD, et al. "More training needed in chronic care: a national survey of family physicians, pediatricians, internists and surgeons," Academic Medicine, June 2004.
4. Johnson JK, Woods DM, Stevens DP, et al. Joy and challenges in improving chronic illness care: capturing daily experiences of academic primary care teams. J Gen Intern Med. 2010;25 Suppl 4:S581–5.

Preface

We are excited. In creating this book, we intend to contribute to a revolution in the structure and delivery of health care. We are referring to "integrated care," care rendered by a multidisciplinary treatment team and prioritizing collaboration between team members [1].

"Comprehensive care," incorporating all components of care required by patients with complex needs, has been described since at least 1980 [2]. In the form of the patient-centered medical home, it has been shown to improve primary medical care and reduce its cost. Well, that is logical, isn't it? If pieces of the medical equation are missing, the results cannot possibly be as good as when they are included. Good care usually also involves the efficient use of medical resources. But, add to that description a precise fit between parts. Treatment components honed, so they work together with precision. With this consideration added, we have *"integrated care."*

Consider, for example, adding a psychiatrist to a treatment team dealing with a critical case of metastatic colon cancer. You have already incorporated oncologists who specialize in the diagnosis and treatment of this particular type of cancer. Next, bring in a member of the clergy if impending death is a consideration and the patient wants spiritual counseling. The medical regimen for the cancer is wearing and painful. It lasts for months and the side effects from both chemotherapy and radiation erode hope and vitality. It is no secret that having psychiatric support and other sources of emotional reinforcement can make all the difference. Consultation among team members is a requirement for success. The team leader needs to be skilled in understanding all the systemic medical and psychiatric requirements of the case and in guiding team members to work with impeccable coordination.

As we see it, there is a difference between "comprehensive" care and "integrated" care. In well-conceived "integrated care," the efficacy of the care reliably exceeds the sum of its parts. Components reinforce each other and do not just add up.

For this book, we have tapped into the "real world" of treatment, the craft of the primary care physician, illustrating how often it functions as a unified, albeit complicated process. This book chronicles the decision making by physicians who take total care of their patients. There is little about this process that has been withheld from the narrative descriptions by the chapter authors. In this book we have included, even emphasized, aspects of the treatment puzzle that are often not considered to be of major significance by treating physicians. These "hidden" factors, however, may play a key role in the success (or failure) of treatment. Complex treatment cases have been deliberately chosen for purposes of illustration. Included are 17 of them. Truthfully, there are few medical cases that are devoid of complexity, but for most of the cases described in this book it is the complexity that leads.

Treatments for cases involving complex patients are the order of the day in much of contemporary medicine. In this book, we illustrate integrated approaches required to effectively treat these complicated patients. We cap our effort with a proposal to formalize integration of medical care through introducing a new diagnostic classification emphasizing systemic medical-psychiatric comorbidity, "clinical complexity," with the hope that it will become recognized and accepted in the medical community. In effect, we will be advocating for the establishment of a new medical specialization dedicated to the assessment and treatment of these cases. In support of this idea, we also encourage the creation of treatment centers exclusively devoted to the treatment of clinically complex cases.

Kentfield, CA, USA
San Francisco, CA, USA
Steven A. Frankel
James A. Bourgeois

References

1. Nielsen M, Buelt L, Patel K, Nichols L. The patient-centered medical home's impact on cost and quality. Review of Evidence, 2014–2015. 2016.
2. American Association of Family Physicians. Website: http://www.aafp.org/home.html. 2017.

Acknowledgments

We are grateful for the persistence and support of all contributing members of our medical group from the Center for Collaborative, Medicine, Psychiatry, and Psychology, and for the unflagging support provided by our team at Springer: Nadina Persaud our editor and guide, Susan Westendorf our production editor, and Kanimozhi Sekar and Anupradhaam Subramonian our production team. Thanks so much to all of you for making this book possible.

Contents

Contributors

James A. Bourgeois, OD, MD, DFAPA, FAPM Department of Psychiatry, Baylor Scott & White Health, Central Texas Division, Temple, TX, USA

Department of Psychiatry, Texas A and M University Health Sciences Center, College of Medicine, Temple, TX, USA

Department of Psychiatry, University of California San Francisco, School of Medicine, San Francisco, CA, USA

Catharine Clark-Sayles, MD, FACP Internal Medicine, Geriatrics, Greenbrae, CA, USA

Lael Duncan, MD Internal Medicine, Coalition for Compassionate Care of California, Sacramento, CA, USA

Wendi Eden Innovative Sleep Centers, Redding, CA, USA

Elizabeth Etemad, MD Family Medicine, Prima Medical Group, Novato, CA, USA

Steven A. Frankel, MD, DFAPA, FAPM Department of Psychiatry, University of California, School of Medicine, San Francisco, CA, USA

Paul Gilbert, MD School of Medicine, University of California, San Francisco, CA, USA

Carla Graf, PhD, RN, GCNS Office of Population Health and Accountable Care, San Francisco, CA, USA

Gina Intinarelli, RN MS PhD University of California School of Nursing Social and Behavioral Sciences, Vice President Department of Population Health University of California, School of Medicine, San Francisco, CA, USA

Office of Population Health and Accountable Care, San Francisco, CA, USA

Alvin Lau, MD University of California School of Medicine, San Mateo, CA, USA

County Federally Qualified Health Center (FQHC), San Mateo, CA, USA

Jan Maisel, MD FAAP University of California Medical Center, San Mateo, CA, USA

Tamalpais Pediatrics, Larkspur, CA, USA

J. Richard Mendius, MD Sutter Pacific Medical Center, Santa Rosa, CA, USA

Thomas W. Miller LightHouse Family Clinic, Ocean Shore, WA, USA

Currently at Innovative Sleep Centers, Aberdeen, WA, USA

David Palestrant, MD Neurology, Critical Care, Kentfield Long Term Acute Care Hospital, Kentfield, CA, USA

Mehrdad Razavi, MD Innovative Sleep Centers, San Rafael, CA, USA

Curtis (Kip) Roebken, MD Kentfield Long Term Acute Care Hospital, Kentfield, CA, USA

Deepak Sreedharan, MD Neurosciences, Sutter Health, Sacramento, CA, USA

Part I
Overview

Chapter 1
Introduction

Steven A. Frankel and James A. Bourgeois

Medicine is challenging, but not necessarily because of the difficulty encountered when treating medical conditions by themselves. Although there is always one or more central systemic medical illness requiring attention, these are typically complicated with and often overshadowed by psychiatric, social, and health systems considerations. You are faced with a virulent case of systemic lupus erythematosus with multisystems involvement, but the patient has lost her job and one of her teen-age children is addicted to street drugs. What disease or social problem should you target first? Although you have a nurse who can assist you, at what point do you personally advocate for this patient? The health system with which she is registered is difficult to access, and subscribers are impeded by rules and bureaucracy from proactively advocating for their own needs.

This book represents the collaborative effort of 16 physicians, all of whom practice in Marin County, California, just north of the Golden Gate Bridge, and five others who are based at the University of California, San Francisco. Two of the authors are advanced practice nurse practitioners, both with years of clinical experience. In creating this book, we wanted to show it "like it is" and thereby do our part to add a relatively neglected perspective to the medical literature. Medicine

S.A. Frankel, MD (✉)
Department of Psychiatry, University of California, School of Medicine, San Francisco, CA, USA
e-mail: saf@stevenfrankelmd.com

J.A. Bourgeois
Department of Psychiatry, Baylor Scott & White Health, Central Texas Division, Temple, TX, USA

Department of Psychiatry, Texas A and M University Health Sciences Center, College of Medicine, Temple, TX, USA

Department of Psychiatry, University of California San Francisco, School of Medicine, San Francisco, CA, USA
e-mail: James.Bourgeois@BSWHealth.org

© Springer International Publishing AG, part of Springer Nature 2018
S.A. Frankel, J.A. Bourgeois (eds.), *Integrated Care for Complex Patients*,
https://doi.org/10.1007/978-3-319-61214-0_1

is an exciting career. There are few other professions that are as challenging and vital as medicine.

Five of us: J. Richard Mendius MD (Neurology), Philip Erdberg PhD and Diane Engelman PhD (Psychology), and Paul Gilbert MD and Steven Frankel MD (General and Child/Adolescent Psychiatry) initiated monthly meetings in 2007. For the past 10 years, we have met once a month for what has become a broadly specialized consultation-discussion group. These discussions have been uniformly riviting, and the notes from our meetings have been incorporated into the case narratives in this book. It was not long before we expanded to our current 16 members and set on our focus: "clinical complexity." Three years ago, James Bourgeois (Professor of Clinical Psychiatry, University of California Medical School, San Francisco) and I decided to create this book.

To begin:

When we were kids, most of us "played doctor." Simple—your tummy hurt and the pretend nurse gave you a pill. But what if your mommy was also sick, or, was mad at your father? Maybe she did not come home last night and was brought in by the police with bruises on her face. Uh oh, a sweet child's story is suddenly getting messy.

Somehow, the biological already got lost from our story. We have been pulled into a social drama. Or maybe that was always an inherent part of the "sickness."

NOW, you are the primary care physician. You went to medical school to learn how to treat illnesses, you know, the kind that are caused by viruses and pathogenic bacteria, and the body's immune mechanisms gone awry. Add to the list broken bones and an occasional emergency surgery performed in the office.

But, what happened to that little girl? She is now 36 years old, and in addition to her systemic medical illnesses, she is plagued by anxiety. In fact, she has visited the ED at her local hospital four times in the past year with panic attacks including "terrible stomach cramps," unrelated to her menstrual period. Multiple diagnostic tests have been negative. Her anxiety disorder keeps her from working, and child protective services has been called by neighbors when they heard vicious screaming in her apartment.

Complex case? You bet. And, who is going to treat it? Already, for this case, we require a primary care physician, gastroenterologist, a gynecologist, and array of child health experts and social workers.

Welcome to the world of contemporary primary care, the place where everything is treated, in spite of the fact that resources including treatment time tend to be scarce. Adding to these challenges, paperwork is abundant, distracting the physician and staff from attending to their patients' presenting medical and social problems.

Playing doctor was fun. Primary care, as it is now practiced, can be grinding.

Currently, primary care has expanded to become "collaborative care" or "integrated care," and the notion of clinical complexity has become commonplace in the medical vocabulary. The goal of the "new" health care is epitomized by the Institute of Healthcare Improvement's much publicized "triple aim." Involved are improved patient satisfaction and health outcomes, together with reduced medical costs [1]. However, much these innovations help to improve care, they are paired with voluminous rules and regulations such as those associated with Medicare, and the newest care delivery model the "accountable care organization" (ACO) has not yet proved to be cost-effective in complex cases where care coordination and close, ongoing attention to the details of the patient's presenting problems care are required [1]. Added to this makeover, direct physician-to-patient and physician-to-physician conversation has generally been replaced by electronic communication. Record keeping involves sitting at a computer terminal and interacting with an electronic medical record (EMR). Getting to know the patient and establishing a relationship is frequently off the priority list.

The intricacies of contemporary medical care for complex cases such as this one are extensive and involve multiple areas of care including those involving the systemic medical, psychological, social, sociological-ethnic, economic, and health systems. The truth is that derangements in any one of these areas may have the biggest impact on the patient's health and welfare. If you are treating multiple sclerosis as the primary medical disease and the patient has just lost his job, what factor do you think will have the greatest influence on his health and sense of well-being?

In this book, we focus on clinical complexity. We bring you details of the work of physicians, the balance of them primary care physicians. We are convinced that treatment, "trees," in the form of algorithms are vital for physicians finding their way through complex medical challenges. We know, however, that these guides cannot be the full answer to successfully unpacking most complex clinical situations because they tend to leave out the filler elements, especially the human ones. These additional considerations, including social, psychological, care delivery, and financial issues, are not likely to be extraneous. Their importance varies from case to case, and changes from point to point within the same case. To see, the "whole forest" (extending the metaphor) requires an integrative, holistic, and dimensional view of the patient and his/her environment, which is why a "case" is usually more complex and layered than just "the patient's illness."

Watch carefully as the skilled practitioners who have contributed the narratives and didactic chapters in this book do real treatment. Consider the ways they have come to formulate and structure their complex cases and note the instruments they have available for this purpose, including clinical screening tools to help them organize clinical data. Think then about the prospect of training specialized physicians to work preferentially with these difficult cases. (Note that we have switched from "difficult or complex patients" to "difficult or complex cases" because a "case" includes the pathogenic aspects of the contributing environment, not just the patient's pathophysiology.) This is the point at which we stop bemoaning the constraints of contemporary models of primary care including the delivery of care for complex cases, and look for ways to improve it.

Further, we will propose a new subspecialization for physicians who work preferentially with complex cases. This, addition to the contemporary medical specialization cadre, is sorely needed given the masses of complex cases encountered by physicians in primary care practice and the high cost of managing these patients. We believe that this group of physicians (perhaps to be called "complexologists" or a similar, distinctive term) will require unique and thematic training, in the form of a postgraduate fellowships dedicated to understanding and treating clinically complex patients [2]. Further, we recommend the establishment of referral centers specifically designed and staffed for treating these complicated, high-cost patients; such institutions could be modeled, for example, as "complexity management centers."

References

1. McWilliams M.J. Cost containment and the tale of care coordination. N Engl J Med. 2016;375:2218–20.
2. Frankel S, Bourgeois J, Erdberg P. Comprehensive care for complex patients: the medical-psychiatric coordinating physician model. Cambridge: Cambridge University Press; 2014.

Chapter 2
Optimized Primary Care for Complex Patients

Steven A. Frankel and James A. Bourgeois

The Setting for Our Work

This book presents the efforts of a group of dedicated, patient-centered physicians, who 10 years ago organized to pool their training and experiences, and meet regularly to discuss patient care challenges and issues of care delivery. They also independently (yet presciently) understood that a major contemporary encumbrance for systems of clinical care delivery is the care of "complex patients" and the associated "complex cases." These are the patients who are "everyone's" patient, yet "no one's" patient. These are patients who "don't get much better and rarely go away." The antidote for their suffering transcends medical specialty. Thus, they cannot be pigeonholed as "internal medicine patients" or "psychiatric patients." As such, a collaborative approach for patient management involving collegial support for and among the treating physicians is an optimum approach.

What follows in this book is for the most part, a realistic description of the management of challenging primary care patients, especially those in community-based

S.A. Frankel, MD (✉)
Department of Psychiatry, University of California, School of Medicine, San Francisco, CA, USA
e-mail: saf@stevenfrankelmd.com

J.A. Bourgeois
Department of Psychiatry, Baylor Scott & White Health, Central Texas Division, ,
Temple, TX, USA

Department of Psychiatry, Texas A and M University Health Sciences Center,
College of Medicine, Temple, TX, USA

Department of Psychiatry, University of California San Francisco, School of Medicine,
San Francisco, CA, USA
e-mail: James.Bourgeois@BSWHealth.org

© Springer International Publishing AG, part of Springer Nature 2018
S.A. Frankel, J.A. Bourgeois (eds.), *Integrated Care for Complex Patients*,
https://doi.org/10.1007/978-3-319-61214-0_2

practice; medical care "on the front lines." By "community-based practice," we are referring to office-based practice outside of major medical center and large HMOs. Community-based physicians generally practice in small- to moderate-sized multi-specialty groups. These are organizations that utilize physicians and other health professions and may provide a spectrum of health care services. Care delivery and financial structures in these organizations take a variety of forms. Uniting them is the patient and the care required to treat his or her illnesses. In this book, we bring you directly into the world of these physicians.

There are 21 contributors to this book, 18 physicians, two advanced practice nurses, and one attorney specializing in health care law. Fourteen of our authors are physicians primarily practicing in the community, one is the physician director of a "long-term acute care" (LTAC) hospital, another who is also a physician directs a program providing end-of-life services, five others are employed at the University of California, San Francisco (UCSF), and one of the narrative authors, although not employed by UCSF, is the Primary Investigator of a multicenter research project at UCSF. Altogether, these authors provide a diversity of perspectives for readers.

Health care systems, in the latter half of the twentieth century, grew exponentially in the United States, becoming more fragmented and complex as the "industrialization" of medical care progressed. Presently, we have various relatively uncoordinated health related systems, both governmental and private, that finance, provide care, and evaluate the efficiency of health services delivery. Prior to World War II, physicians and nurses provided the bulk of care in hospitals and private medical practices. During and post-World War II, however, employers became the largest financiers of health care by contracting with insurers. However, this trend is now changing, as the cost burden is being shifted to employees and large employers are managing health insurance costs more defensively.

We now have a multiplicity of clinicians from various professional disciplines as well as other medical and administrative personnel involved in patient care. The mix is particularly varied for complex cases. The systems in which clinicians now practice are largely uncoordinated and loosely linked with other systems, creating duplication, inconsistency, and increased costs for patient services. Patients are more mobile and have less employer loyalty or opportunity available to remain in stable employment situations. The consequence is the increased frequency of changes in insurance and longer periods of noninsurance. This instability can readily diminish or destroy the relationship between a primary care provider and patient.

Most front line medical care is provided by primary care physicians (PCPs). Although their training in general medicine overlaps, they also frequently have areas of focus based on additional training and experience. These physicians are in a sense the "gatekeepers" of the U.S. medical system. The medical scope of internal medicine and family medicine are in many ways similar, but internal medicine training emphasizes in-depth familiarity with disease entities, whereas family medicine is characterized by comprehensiveness, familiarity with a broad range of disease, and also management of some OB/GYN and pediatric care, which are not typical in internal medicine practices. Physicians from both specialties are dedicated to the delivery of excellent medical care, but may see themselves as having somewhat different missions.

Primary Care

The Institute of Medicine (IOM) has developed a commonly accepted definition of primary care: "Primary care is the provision of integrated, accessible health care services by clinicians who are accountable for addressing a large majority of personal health care needs, developing a sustained partnership with patients, and practicing in the context of family and community." The term "integrated" in the IOM definition encompasses "the provision of comprehensive, coordinated, and continuous services that provide a seamless process of care" [1].

The American Academy of Family Physicians further defines primary care as, "Primary care is that care provided by physicians specifically trained for and skilled in comprehensive first contact and continuing care for persons with any undiagnosed sign, symptom, or health concern not limited by problem origin (biological, behavioral, or social), organ system, or diagnosis. A primary care practice serves as the patient's first point of entry into the health care system and as the continuing focal point for all needed health care services. Primary care practices provide patients with ready access to their own personal physician, or to an established back-up physician when the primary physician is not available. Primary care physicians generally devote the majority of their practice to providing services to a defined population of patients. The style of primary care practice is such that the personal primary care physician serves as the entry point for substantially all of the patient's medical and health care needs..."[2].

Primary care physicians are patient advocates in coordinating the use of the health care system to benefit the patient. Primary care specialties include family medicine, general internal medicine, obstetrics and gynecology, and general pediatrics. There are other clinicians, who render primary care, typically under the supervision of and/or consultation with a physician. Such clinicians include nurse practitioners and physician assistants.

The delivery of medical care is costly, and the challenge of delivering technically excellent care with input from required medical specialists and access to complex laboratory and diagnostic imaging as well as other technology, generally exceeds the capability of an individual practitioner or even the resources of a multidisciplinary group. The alternative is care where costs and referrals are managed through contracts with larger, more financially capable organizations, that is, "managed care."

Managed Care

Contrasting to traditional private practice is managed care. Managed care is available as a network of services. In managed care, as it is conceived, the cost of and access to treatment is regulated by a managing company. The objective of managed care is to provide regulated medical services on a broad scale and thereby reduce the cost of providing health benefits and improve access to care. In choosing managed care, patients typically agree to use a designated group of physicians and hospitals.

Managed care in the United States was introduced by the Health Maintenance Organization Act of 1973. A Health Maintenance Organization (HMO) is a coordinated delivery system that combines both the financing and delivery of health care for enrollees. Services provided by HMOs are generally organized as follows. Each member is assigned a "gatekeeper," generally a primary care physician (PCP). All health care services are authorized by that physician. Nonemergent hospital admissions generally require preauthorization initiated and/or coordinated by the PCP. HMOs may contract with insurers. This arrangement contrasts with traditional fee-for-service ("indemnity") where in exchange for a paid premium, an insurance company pays fees for each service provided to an insured patient. Fee-for-service plans offer a wide choice of doctors and hospitals. Basic protection provides partial or full reimbursement for the costs of a hospital room, hospital services, care and supplies, cost of surgery in or out of hospital, and provider visits.

Alternative managed care structures include independent practice associations (IPAs) and preferred provider organizations (PPOs). An independent practice association (IPA) is a legal entity that contracts with a group of physicians. Most often, the physicians are paid on a basis of capitation, a set amount of reimbursement per unit time for each enrolled person assigned to that physician or group of physicians. Because of its group structure, PPO membership allows a discount below regularly charged fee-for-service rates of the designated providers partnered with the organization. Unlike an HMO plan, which has a copayment cost share feature, a PPO generally does not have a copay and instead has a deductible and coinsurance feature. The deductible must be paid in full before any benefits are provided. After the deductible is met, the coinsurance requirements apply.

A point-of-service plan (POS) utilizes some of the features of both of the above plans with benefit levels varying and depending on whether one receives care in or out of the health insurance company's network of providers. A participant may receive care from non-network providers but usually with significant out-of-pocket costs. Participants may also be responsible for co-payments, coinsurance and an annual deductible. There are levels of progressively higher patient financial participation as the patient moves away from the more managed features of the plan.

Community-Based Primary Care

Community-based primary care physicians practicing alone or in small-to-moderate-sized groups work in the "trenches" and generally do so by choice. These physicians are characteristically focused on treating their individual patients. They may treat individual patients over years. They frequently have chosen community practice outside the HMO or major medical center to deliver care as they believe it "should be done." These relatively independent physicians confront several types of complexity in the work they do. In addition to patient (clinical) complexity, there are complex rules governing the availability of resources, complexity in managing and collaborating with the personnel who render care, and complex challenges to the ongoing implementation of care. Frequently added are the problems associated with of securing adequate reimbursement for services. Exacting financial regulations and an often unfriendly medical–legal climate complete the list.

In this book, you will find 16 clinical narratives involving complex cases managed mainly in primary care with consultative assistance from specialty physicians and allied health professionals. These narratives are modified to protect the privacy of the involved patients. They highlight the illnesses experienced by these patients, the social and administrative complexity confronted when treating them, and their clinical outcomes. Based on the collective experience of our group, the Center for Medicine, Psychiatry, and Psychology (CMPP), in Kentfield California, we propose a model of "integrated/specialty-supported comprehensive primary care" that we believe is preferable for the management of complex patients and the associated complex cases. This model preserves the centrality of the physician–patient relationship as the "therapeutic keystone" to optimizing treatment of these frequently chronically and comorbidly ill patients. We are also aware that in this era of multi-specialty group-based outpatient care that patients' loyalty may be to a group of clinicians with whom they have regular contact rather than to an individual physician.

More complex medical systems such as academic medical centers and HMOs, although having in-house access to primary care physicians and specialists as well as other health practitioners, may not necessarily be designed to optimally support primary care physicians in personally managing these complex patients. Health care systems responsible for managing large cohorts of complex patients may benefit from the organically developed, patient-centered model we describe [3]. This book, written in the tradition of narrative medicine, is intended to be read by physicians, other clinicians, medical administrators, patients, and anyone else who is interested in what physicians and their support staff actually do. We especially emphasize the physician–patient relationship as a fundamental source of efficacy when working in complex clinical situations.

Medicine on the "Front Lines"

The following is a patient-centered snapshot of medical practice as it exists outside of the highly systematized and regulated world of the HMO or major medical center. Start with Ms. A., a prototypical patient who comes to your office referred by a relative. From the start, she inherently both trusts and distrusts you. It is usually that way. You are the "elevated" doctor charged with providing a "cure" for her by now multiple sources of pain and disability. However, after the first several appointments, Ms. A. finds herself suspecting that you have "missed something" because her medical condition "does not seem to be improving." Maybe you did not take a good enough history or order the proper laboratory tests. Maybe you are not clever enough to help her. These judgments are typical, and may at times be accurate. After all, no one completely trusts another person, physician or otherwise, right from the start and providing medical care for chronic conditions can be a high stakes challenge.

Fortunately, over time, you and Ms. A. develop a comfortable working relationship. But, behind the scenes, all may not be so sanguine and her dissatisfaction may again work its way to the surface. Ms. A. needs an MRI to help clarify the source of her abdominal pain. However, her insurance company requires preauthorization for the procedure. The forms are filled out and submitted, but the request is denied. Or, maybe Ms. A. has not met her deductible for the year and she has a "high deductible policy" meaning that she will have significant out-of-pocket costs even for a covered procedure. After the procedure, a large bill arrives. Ms. A. cannot help but feel that you and your staff have not been looking out for her welfare. In either case, Ms. A. concludes that, you, the physician, could have "done better."

How could Ms. A. know that behind the scenes, your office staff has been making extended—albeit unsuccessful—telephone calls to her insurance company attempting to secure approval and payment for the MRI. The request is denied for a second time. In this case, the patient did not "fall within the guidelines" for approval of an MRI for her set of symptoms." Already, after only a few office visits, you and Ms. A. are faced with a multitude of care associated complexities, including diagnostic, interpersonal, and insurance-based challenges, all potentially eroding the effectiveness of the medical care she receives. The "moral of the story?" It is great to commit yourself to deliver the best care, but successfully managing the constant administrative hassles and denials and still coming out "on top" is another matter.

Adding to the complications of delivering adequate primary care for complex patients are communication issues. Communication is a costly commodity in medicine because of the time required. Physicians and allied health personnel are increasingly forced to rely on electronic medical records (EMR) and digital communications requiring them to spend significant part of clinical appointments at a computer screen. While this development results in more reliable and accessible patient health records, greater administrative efficiency, and improved patient safety, maintaining a robust physician–patient relationship in this context often becomes more challenging. Face-to-face time with patients is charateristically reduced. Live collaborative discussions among physicians are likely also to be sacrificed, with email rather that phone conversations becoming the preferred means of communication.

In this book, you will see how primary care physicians (PCPs) on the front lines manage care–associated problems such as these, as well as administrative roadblocks limiting access to clinical resources.[1] Our objective is to explore the realities of medical care for complex cases, especially in the world beyond the medical center and HMO. Central to this work are primary care physicians and their relationships with physician specialists and health care facilities.

---

[1] "PCP" is also used as an abbreviation for "primary care provider". In this book, we will restrict its use to "primary care physician"

Our Group: The Center for Collaborative Medicine, Psychiatry, and Psychology

Physicians are busy, often too busy to spend time conferring with one another. In 2007, several physicians from our community began to address this problem by establishing a forum for discussing clinical problems and identifying better ways to manage the complex clinical dilemmas they routinely encountered in their practices. The original group coalesced around internal medicine, family medicine, pediatrics, and psychiatry. Specialists in neurology, pain medicine, sleep medicine, immunology, and an advanced practice nurse were soon added. All of our physicians are board certified in at least one medical specialty. We have been further supported by a psychologist-statistician and a neuropsychologist who consult to us. We are very aware of the critical role of allied professionals who facilitate and sustain our work and have since been joined by a second advanced practice nurse who is an expert on care delivery systems.

We meet monthly to discuss cases and practice-related concerns, always fascinated by the clinical persistence and creativity of our fellow group members. Although constrained by many of the same stringent controls on quality of care and resources encountered in highly structured care organizations such as HMOs and major medical centers, community-based practice is often characterized by greater freedom to creatively organize and manage clinical work. The case narratives in this book illustrate that assertion. Our group discussions are always pointedly patient-centered. By meeting regularly, we maintain our resolve not to let our clinical judgment become distracted by the multiple roadblocks encountered in our daily practices. We have all been impressed by how faithfully the our group members adhere to the principles of the Hippocratic Oath, all providing the most effective available treatments while maintaining compassion and therapeutic humility. This stance is typically sustained in the face of financial sacrifice and challenging time demands.

The notion of a treatment alliance should hardly be foreign to any reader with a medical background. Not long ago, it was considered to be the cornerstone of medical practice. To the extent that it can persist within the time demands, legal regulations, and financial constraints of contemporary medicine, it lives on as such in the minds of physicians and especially those in primary care practice. In primary care practice conducted with this spirit, your physician is likely to think of you as "his or her patient," and breaches in the continuity of that relationship are likely to be considered disruptive to patient care, especially in the face of complex clinical challenges.

Especially with complex patients and related complex cases, the physician–patient relationship over time remains the central therapeutic tool in many of these cases and is rarely missing from the others. This is especially so when the involvement of multiple specialists does not itself lead to definitive, disease-curing care and the main therapeutic task is accomplishment of functional optimization, especially given the coping limitations resulting from chronic illness. This idea will be more fully developed in subsequent chapters and is exemplified in the case narratives, each containing reflections by the narrative's author.

References

1. Institute of Medicine (IOM). In: Donaldson MS, Yordy KD, Lohr KN, Vanselow NA, editors. Primary care: America's health in a new era. Washington, DC: National Academy Press; 1996.
2. American Association of Family Physicians. Website: http://www.aafp.org/home.html; 2017.
3. Frankel S, Bourgeois J, Erdberg P. Comprehensive care for complex patients: the medical-psychiatric coordinating physician model. Cambridge: Cambridge University Press; 2014.

Chapter 3
Clinical Complexity: The Challenge of Complexity in Medical Practice

Steven A. Frankel and James A. Bourgeois

An encouraging phrase: "integrated care," the combined management of a patient's systemic medical and psychiatric illnesses. However, add to this picture psychological and social difficulties, as well as problems getting healthcare needs met and complexity moves to the forefront [1]. Patients with a mixture of these afflictions and complicated personal needs are "clinically complex." With these patients as the target group, integrated care has come to the fore as a pressing topic in contemporary care delivery.

Currently, "Collaborative Care," pioneered at the University of Washington's AIMS Center, is a highly visible model for organization and delivery of integrated care [2]. In addition to PCP primary care ownership, collaborative care ordinarily includes systematic medical and psychiatric assessments that involve symptom screenings with standardized psychiatric rating scales for diagnostic and monitoring purposes. In collaborative care programs for depression, for example, a validated and structured depression assessment tool such as the Patient Health Questionnaire-9 (PHQ-9) is part of routine clinical visits, both for initial case finding and diagnosis and measuring treatment outcome. These assessments are usually done by a care manager who may be a nurse, social worker, or other health

S.A. Frankel, MD (✉)
Department of Psychiatry, University of California, School of Medicine,
San Francisco, CA, USA
e-mail: saf@stevenfrankelmd.com

J.A. Bourgeois
Department of Psychiatry, Baylor Scott & White Health, Central Texas Division,
Temple, TX, USA

Department of Psychiatry, Texas A and M University Health Sciences Center,
College of Medicine, Temple, TX, USA

Department of Psychiatry, University of California San Francisco, School of Medicine,
San Francisco, CA, USA
e-mail: James.Bourgeois@BSWHealth.org

© Springer International Publishing AG, part of Springer Nature 2018
S.A. Frankel, J.A. Bourgeois (eds.), *Integrated Care for Complex Patients*,
https://doi.org/10.1007/978-3-319-61214-0_3

professional. That person also provides a coordinating role including longitudinal symptom monitoring and algorithm-based treatment interventions for the comorbid psychiatric illnesses; e.g., major depression and generalized anxiety disorder, identified by these screening instruments. Psychiatric and related systemic medical consultation is typically provided by a psychiatrist who can make recommendations for additional interventions [3]. Specialty referral is available for the most complex patients and those who are treatment failures according to standardized practice algorithms.

The following is a brief case example from the Perspective of a Primary Care physician providing treatment.

You've gone to great lengths to determine why Mr. B., age 73, keeps developing unexplained infections. He apparently has an unusual immunodeficiency disorder that may be an effect of lisinopril he takes to regulate his blood pressure. In rare cases, lisinopril can cause bone marrow depression, hemolytic anemia, neutropenia, and thrombocytopenia [4]. Mr. B. also suffers from osteoporosis and last year he received a "watch and wait" recommendation for stage 2 prostate adenocarcinoma. All these conditions should be readily manageable medically. A major personal complication, however, is that Mr. B. has just lost his wife. He is also drinking excessively and is unwilling and perhaps unable to get adequate treatment for this. So what clinical components should you target in this situation and in what sequence? How to integrate the pieces into a rational treatment plan? This is the type of situation that the clinician authors of this book face daily. Daunting? You bet! And always with problematical consequences for oversights and mistakes as they impact the patient's quality of life and even survival.

It's not hard to understand what integrated care should consist of in this case. Mr. B.'s alcohol use disorder will need immediate attention. He will, of course, require psychiatric care, most likely involving psychotherapy and psychotropic medication. Grief counseling probably should be added. He needs referral to an immunologist to see if the cause of his immunological deficiency is being properly diagnosed and treated, and to a urologist for management of his prostate cancer. The osteoporosis is not of immediate concern, but could ultimately contribute to an orthopedic crisis such as a hip fracture. Add that a "nonmedical" factor significantly burdening Mr. B's health situation is his intense preoccupation with his cancer. He is unwilling to be reassured that this particular type of cancer generally has a good prognosis, and he focuses on it to the exclusion of managing his more urgent medical concerns.

Technically, Mr. B.'s case requires attention to all the care-related dimensions mentioned as constituting clinical complexity: systemic medical, psychiatric, psychological-social, and health systems availability. Mr. B. has several illnesses including one, his hematological disorder, that has vexed his treating physicians. However, the knowledge and resources are available to address all of these. It is the personal factors, however, that mainly impede treatment. Mr. B. is pathologically anxious about his cancer, distracting him from attending to other pertinent health concerns. His personal life has also been disrupted by loss of his wife. Adequate treatment for his alcohol dependence is lacking.

How to maintain a useful focus for care in this situation? Who should and can provide treatment? Is it reasonable to rely on a PCP to deal with all these problems, directly or through care coordination? To what extent should medical specialists be involved? A care manager's presence is called for but may not be available depending on the model of care delivery available to him.

How Much Primary and How Much Specialty Care?

Welcome to the challenge of primary care. Here, the physician reflexively takes on most comers. However, there are mounting restrictions on available resources by government and private insurers, and these have been introduced in spite of increased patient flow (in the USA in part due to the Affordable Care Act leading to increased access to health insurance). To treat "everyone," these physicians need to make choices and in so doing must restrict the time spent with patients or allocate care to clinicians such as nurse practitioners or physician assistants.

As medicine has become technologically more sophisticated it has also become more specialized. The American Association of Medical Colleges lists 120 medical specialties and subspecialties [5]. While specialties and subspecialties have been created in response to advances in medical knowledge, excessive reliance on them runs the risk of fragmenting basic medical care, with specialists and primary care physicians often practicing in different locations and impeded by communication challenges.

We already have a variety of topics complicating the work of primary care physicians. Included are the complexity of many of the treatment situations they encounter. Added are the extra burdens imposed by chronic illnesses including (1) infirmities of advancing age, (2) fragmentation of care with specialists practicing in relatively isolated "silos" and for the most part communicating mainly electronically, (3) specialization itself moved forward by advancement of medical science toward "precision medicine," and (4) strain on PCPs imposed by upward spiraling medical costs and the resulting need to conserve healthcare resources.

How to correct this imbalance between primary and specialty care and achieve a desirable and affordable integration? It is tempting to allocate a large share of the work to primary care physicians, moving PCPs back toward their roles from before clinical specialization became the rule. But in that case, what to do about the advanced training and technical sophistication required to practice modern medicine, e.g., the background and skill needed to diagnose and treat esoteric aspects of Mr. B.'s immunodeficiency? As a PCP do you simply do your best to manage challenging clinical situations without substantial specialty/subspecialty support or do you engage specialists as possible?

Historical Perspective

While often underappreciated, complex patients and cases are an epidemic of contemporary times. This development is explained by several convergent factors. Until the twentieth century, epidemic infectious diseases were a major source of limited life expectancy. Before the 1920s, juvenile onset diabetes mellitus was typically rapidly fatal. In recent decades, remarkable progress has occurred in oncology, internal medicine, surgery, and neurology. Mortality and morbidity from cancer, cardiovascular (CV) disease, and stroke (CVA) have been reduced. While these diseases remain important public health problems, they are now more manageable and often preventable. AIDS (HIV), a disease once nearly uniformly fatal, has been transformed in 30 years to a chronic disease, usually treatable with medication. Advances in psychopharmacology have significantly improved the potential for improved functional prognosis for patients with schizophrenia, bipolar disorder, major depression, and panic disorder. Added to this trend are other shifts from "acutely lethal" illnesses to "chronic survivable" ones. Paradoxically, however, the public burden of disease has not decreased. With people in many parts of the world living longer, the number of chronically ill and complex patients has increased.

Complex Patients and Complex Cases

What complex patients typically have in common is chronic systemic illness and comorbid psychiatric illness, often including substance use disorder and social problems. Their social problems may include disrupted relationships, as well as housing, financial, insurance difficulties, and, finally, clinical services access difficulties. Substance use disorder, so common in this group, is a psychiatric illness that is often phenomenologically and administratively separated from the rest of psychiatry. For the most part, it is treated behaviorally and is distinguished by its tenacity and frequent comorbidity with personality disorder.

Inasmuch as patients live life as an integrated experience, they cannot be expected to cleanly separate their "medical" from "social" needs. This tendency toward "lumping" results in patients seeking "medical" interventions for problems which are fundamentally "personal" or "social." Witness a patient who is repeatedly brought to the emergency department (ED) for recurrent abdominal pain for which no identifiable cause can be found or a dementia patient who, despite being herself clinically stable, is taken to the ED due to her response to a loss of a stable social placement.

Sub-categories of Clinical Complexity

Diagnostic Complexity: The definition of clinical complexity can be expanded. In many situations medical complexity secondarily includes psychiatric comorbidity. Within this group are patients with disabling somatic complaints for which there are little or no objective physical, laboratory, or diagnostic imaging findings. In others this relationship is reversed, and a predominantly psychiatric presentation is complicated by systemic medical illness. We refer to complex patients with diagnostic challenges as "diagnostically complex." Diagnostically complex patients are commonly encountered in medical services of major medical centers.

Operational Complexity and Management Complexity: Further broadening the definition of clinical complexity are the designations "operational complexity" and "management complexity." "Operational complexity" refers to a treatment effort requiring committed collaboration among multiple clinicians who may or may not be organized into a treatment team. "Management complexity" refers to patients whose clinical management is particularly challenging, for example, as a result of a comorbid personality disorder and substance abuse. These are often referred to as "difficult patients" [6–8]. In emergency departments they are often called "frequent flyers." They usually overutilize resources ("hyperutilizers") and elude attempts to manage their care efficiently. Their care is often characterized by breaches in the treatment that may include non-compliant behavior with added threats of malpractice litigation.

There is value in distinguishing a "medically complex patient" from a "complex case." A complex patient may be someone with complex systemic medical and psychiatric illness but limited interpersonal entanglements. In the least problematic version, that patient might have an acceptable level of clinical engagement, basic communication skills, and show an adherence to treatment. For the designation to be expanded to "complex case," the patient needs to present with a significant mixture of behavioral, social, and/or care delivery challenges. Behaviorally, such a patient may show any of the following: poor adherence to treatment, maladaptive acting out behavior, a tendency to crisis presentations, poor access to insurance and other financial backing, and inadequate social support generally with problematic entanglements with others. Strictly speaking, a complex case may or may not be focused around a medically complex patient.

Convergent with the recognition of the urgent need to attend to complex cases is the staggering costs complex patients and related cases accrue. According to one source, complex patients constitute approximately 5% of the patient population and use about 50% of health resources [9]. Health plans can readily identify these "high utilizers," a term that is often synonymous with complex patients, based on data analysis identifying excessive clinical encounters over time. Noble efforts in the USA, motivated by the Affordable Care Act, to increase efficiency of healthcare services delivery are at best challenged, if not frankly threatened if these who are conducting these projects do not explicitly come up with ways to manage complex patients' excessive and inappropriate resource utilization.

The challenge of complex patients and cases, especially given how ubiquitous these are and how their multiple needs conflict with the current organization of healthcare into relatively isolated "silos," should be clear by this point. These patients need fully coordinated care and, at the same time, behavior regulation to manage their frequent tendency to be indiscriminate in their use of provider time and other resources. Identifying these patients and then treating them, whether with supportive or curative treatments, is a major medical and economic task at this time.

From this point through Chaps. 4, 5, and 6 we move to established and proposed models for treating this population of patients.

References

1. Kathol R, Gatteau S. Healing mind and body: a critical issue for health care reform. Westport: Preager; 2007.
2. AIMS Center, University of Washington. Website: https://aims.uw.edu/.
3. Huffman JC, Niazi SK, Rundell JR, Sharpe M, Katon WJ. Essential articles on collaborative care models for the treatment of psychiatric disorders in medical settings: a publication by the academy of psychosomatic medicine research and evidence-based practice committee. Psychosomatics. 2014;55(2):109–22.
4. Medline Plus, National Laboratory of Medicine.
5. American Association of Medical Colleges. Website 2017. https://www.aamc.org/cim/specialty/exploreoptions/list/.
6. Frankel S, Bourgeois J, Erdberg P. Comprehensive Care for Complex Patients: the medical-psychiatric coordinating physician model. Cambridge: Cambridge University Press; 2013.
7. de Jonge P, Huyse FJ, Stiefel FC. Case and care complexity in the medically ill. Med Clin North Am. 2006;90(4):679–92.
8. Kathol RG, Perez R, Cohen J. The integrated case management manual: assisting complex patients regain physical and mental health. New York: Springer; 2010.
9. Kathol RG, Lattimer C, Gold G, Perez R, Gutteridge D. Creating clinical and economic "wins" through integrated case management lessons for physicians and health system administrators. Prof Case Manag. 2011;16(6):290–8.

Chapter 4
Models for Managing Complex Cases in Both Inpatient and Outpatient Settings

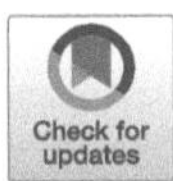

Steven A. Frankel and James A. Bourgeois with Colin Leary

Models of integrated, multispecialty treatment for complex clinical cases have evolved as the awareness of the ubiquity of such cases and their cost to the medical system has grown. Traditionally, primary care physicians focused mainly on treating systemic medical illness. Generally these treatments had a dyadic (patient-primary care physician) or triadic (patient-primary care physician-specialist physician) structure. The patient's overall care was "owned" by the primary care physician, and the physician-patient relationship was the basis of the clinical interaction. Allied health personnel such as physician assistants or nurses were regularly involved in patient care, but the physician remained central to the treatment relationship.

Newer treatment models appropriate for treating complex cases tend to be comprehensive, emphasizing coordination of medical services through multidisciplinary patient care teams. With "integrated care," the targeted pathology is generally comorbid illness, frequently consisting of combined systemic medical-psychiatric illness, but also nonmedical conditions with a psychological and/or social basis. Coordination of these treatments may be led by allied health personnel who share

S.A. Frankel, MD (✉)
Department of Psychiatry, University of California, School of Medicine, San Francisco, CA, USA
e-mail: saf@stevenfrankelmd.com

J.A. Bourgeois
Department of Psychiatry, Baylor Scott & White Health, Central Texas Division, Temple, TX, USA

Department of Psychiatry, Texas A and M University Health Sciences Center, College of Medicine, Temple, TX, USA

Department of Psychiatry, University of California San Francisco, School of Medicine, San Francisco, CA, USA
e-mail: James.Bourgeois@BSWHealth.org

C. Leary
University of California Medical Center, San Francisco

responsibly for patient care with a primary care physician. For these treatments a physician or, depending on the local jurisdiction, another clinician with medical training such as a nurse practitioner, almost always has ultimate responsibility for planning and directing patient care. One model designated for the most difficult to treat patients with severe systemic medical and psychiatric pathology, "the Medical-Psychiatric Coordinating Physician Model" (MPCP), has a psychiatrist in charge of coordinating and leading all treatment activities for highly complex patients with comorbid systemic medical and psychiatric illness [1]. In highly structured settings such as HMOs or in academic medical centers, a wide range of other models may be adopted to fit with patient needs and institutional goals and resources.

The experience of treating complex patients with the typicality of systemic medical illness, psychiatric comorbidity, and personal-social problems, is in alignment with the "biopsychosocial model" [2]. Attention to these three parameters increases the probability of an optimized treatment outcome as more contributing factors are taken into consideration. This term refers both to the patient experience of illness and the clinician management of the same array of illnesses. Encompassed are the variable contributions from biological (physical source of disease), psychological (the patients' internal psychological experience of disease and other stressors), and social (the impact of illness within the patient's social situation, including care access) sources. It is important to recall that psychiatric interventions (e.g., psychotherapy) may be applied broadly to address social as well as psychiatric illness-specific matters (e.g., family focused therapy) so that outpatient mental health care goes far beyond merely "managing psychiatric illness."

Management of Complex Cases: Institutional Settings

Large medical center settings offer advantages for the identification and treatment of complex patients and cases. They also may have fundamental disadvantages. In this chapter we start by discussing the advantages.

Most large medical center settings such as academic medical centers and HMOs depend on case management to support clinical work with complex cases. Case managers may come from a variety of disciplines and include nurses, social workers, care managers, and patient "navigators." In institutional settings for outpatient care, comprehensive outpatient care programs serving complex cases may include:

(a) "Disease management" models.[1]

---

[1] "Disease management" is a system of coordinated health-care interventions and communications for populations with conditions in which patient self-care efforts are emphasized. The "disease management model" utilizes teams of nurses and care managers who may assess patients over the phone. Disease management efforts include regular assessment of known patient populations to identify subtle changes that could affect their overall state of health. Early identification of changes allows involved clinicians to guide self-care interventions, containing the need for more extensive medical intervention.

(b) "Patient-centered medical homes" where a physician is in charge of a multidisciplinary team.
(c) Other models of care such as collaboratively administered "stepped care" where patients are referred successively to increasingly appropriate levels of care [3].
(d) Modern clinics may have on-site embedded psychiatric and other mental health services for the management of psychiatric comorbidity within the medical clinic. Such services optimally include social workers (MSWs), or care managers for management of social, housing, insurance, and other external problems that complicate efficient care delivery.
(e) In addition, the primary medical team may order referrals for supportive and complementary clinical services e.g., ongoing psychotherapy and substance use disorder treatment that are not typically provided within the medical clinic.
(f) Patients with severe chronic psychiatric illness, for whom psychiatric illnesses are the primary source of clinical complexity and who are prone to psychiatric decompensation, are often best served in a psychiatric specialty clinic. Examples include patients with schizophrenia, bipolar disorder, or borderline personality disorder. These clinics have psychiatric illness as their primary focus. Systemic medical care may be offered on the premises or separately.

Management of complex patients and cases within these larger systems of care can be optimized by a comprehensive electronic medical record (EMR) and review system where all clinical care is documented and can be communicated centrally. Complex patients are usually identified by their hyper-utilization of clinical services, and their seeking of health-care services significantly in excess of those of typical patients. They are also particularly likely to use the emergency department (ED), use excessive medical specialty resources, and have higher than average number of inpatient admissions.

One method for accomplishing a review of this sort is through complex case review teams. A multidisciplinary team with representatives from general internal medicine, psychiatry, pharmacy, social work, nursing, and other health-care personnel meets periodically in a case registry review session. Each of the hyper-utilizing patients (typically defined by the medical care delivery system as requiring excessive and often clinically inappropriate use of various clinical services) is presented at team meetings where all of their clinical encounters per unit time are examined by the team. The physician members of the team offer input regarding medical workup results and medical management. This method is successfully used by us at the University of California, San Francisco in a clinical service devoted to evaluating and treating complex patients/cases [4]. Many of these patients will be found to have suboptimally managed psychiatric illness, and recommendations of the psychiatric consultant are sought. Comprehensive medication review by the clinical pharmacist and team physicians can lead to medication streamlining, minimization or discontinuation of unneeded or potentially harmful medications, and plans for optimized laboratory monitoring of medications. For patients with evidence of poor compliance with outpatient clinic attendance and, as is often the case, corresponding inappropriate use of the ED as a substitute source of primary care, assignment of a case manager and/or health-care navigator to facilitate appropriate use of services and adherence is accomplished. Social work interventions (alternatively carried out by case managers) are also offered for social, family support, and social systems problems. These team recommendations are then shared with the patient's primary care physician (PCP) for implementation.

Of note, complex patients pose financial and clinical challenges for accountable care organizations (ACOs) and other care delivery structures where the care institution is clinically and financially responsible for total medical services to enrolled patients. Laudable endeavors to make clinical care more efficient for the total population of care enrollees can themselves be put at risk by the hyper-utilization of complex patients. Hence, institutions contemplating adoption of an ACO are advised to a priori explore models of care specifically tailored for and targeted at complex patients early in the process of creating the ACO.

Management of Complex Cases: Community Primary Care Settings

Complex cases are ubiquitous in outpatient settings. A PCP is generally the central physician, with specialty care routed through and coordinated by that PCP. Accomplished within a primary care consultation model, this method offers the advantages of active collaboration between the PCP and medical consultants. For those cases with comorbid psychiatric illness, psychiatric symptom rating scales (e.g., PHQ-9, GAD-7, MoCA) are routinely used. Primary care for these patients can be supported by psychiatric consultation along with social work and/or case management, when available. Psychiatric referral is utilized for the more complex psychiatric illnesses. Other mental health personnel who can be integrated into primary care include psychologists, psychiatric nurse practitioners, psychiatric social workers, and case managers.

Management of psychiatric illness using symptom rating scales and outcome monitoring may result in improved outcomes and less inappropriate use of general medical services. The psychiatric consultant as part of his/her role assesses and manages psychiatric issues including substance use disorders, while offering behavioral management advice. Detailed understanding of the needs of complex patients may, however, be incomplete when using only the screening-based psychiatric treatment algorithms. Complex patients are often characterized by their multiple psychiatric comorbidities, often the "tri-morbidity" of depressive disorder, substance use disorder, and personality disorder. As such, they may benefit from early recognition of psychiatric pathology and referral for psychiatric consultation where their complex psychiatric needs can be fully evaluated and addressed. With acknowledgment that these patients are unlikely to become entirely "well" and move to becoming "low" utilizers, a pragmatic, albeit intermediate, goal for their care is to use more primary care and psychiatric support and less emergency department, hospital, or other medical specialty care. Behavioral goals may include those set by Medicare or insurance payors, for example, tracking days absent from work.

Optimized Management of Complex Patients in Outpatient Settings

Optimized management of complex patients in a primary care model could operate like this. The PCP would have an intrinsic interest in the management of complex patients. This physician would need to accept that complex patients are not likely to be "cured" of their illnesses. The goal, rather, is to manage the case, optimize functional status, minimize the risks of iatrogenic illness, and, in effect, consider "complexity itself as the equivalent of a chronic illness." The patient should have regular, scheduled, predictable appointments with the physician so that the visits are not "triggered" by acute symptom presentations. The physician should seek to focus maximally on one or two problems per visit, and assess function, not symptoms, as the primary outcome measures. The primary care physician should optimally be comfortable with pragmatic psychiatric techniques such as behavioral activation, CBT, and supportive psychotherapy approaches such as encouragement of efforts at active coping (defined in observable behavioral terms) in the face of illness, doubting, or dysphoria. The physician should minimize the use of high-risk medications (e.g., anticholinergics, steroids, benzodiazepines, opioids) unless explicitly indicated for a particular illness in an evidence-based way. Depressive and anxiety disorders are common in complex patients, and clinical psychopharmacologic intervention either by the PCP or the psychiatrist should be tied to symptom rating scales for outcome monitoring. These treatments and goals are practical and in accord with behavioral techniques, useable in primary care offices, and separate from the in-depth psychiatric assessment and treatment that less responsive cases may require.

Psychiatric Consultation in a Complex Case Treatment Model

When psychiatric management is beyond the scope of the PCP, referrals for higher levels of psychiatric care should be facilitated. Ideally, psychiatric consultation should be readily available within this model and reciprocal communication between the PCP and psychiatrist regularly established. It is a common fallacy among physicians to view outpatient psychiatric care as limited to "medication management." The psychiatric consultant is critical in explicating the nature and extent of the patient's psychiatric comorbid illness(es), including substance use disorders and neurocognitive disorders. When psychotropic medications are prescribed, they need to fit into the patient's overall medication profile. Other functions of the psychiatric consultant include instruction in achieving desirable behavior such as adherence with appointments, compliance with treatment, appropriate use of primary care, and reduction in the inappropriate use of the ED and hospital.

Social Evaluation

Complex patients should also routinely have a complete social assessment. Additional assessment of the often associated psychological and social problems that complicate the patients' presentation is essential and is an excellent role for non-physician mental health clinicians. This evaluation is often efficiently accomplished by a nurse or physician assistant. Included in the assessment should be an evaluation of the patient's social situation (e.g., housing, transportation, social support, relationships) and insurance/disability issues. Supportive counseling can be provided on these matters, accomplishing "social systems engineering" and facilitating social stability.

Examples of Complex Care Models

Of note, there are settings offering comprehensive care that utilize elements of the model explicated above. HIV care models and cancer centers are two examples. These programs deviate somewhat from the above model for primary care treatment of complex cases. They are illness specific and thus not "generically" associated with primary care, but, because of their disease management focus, do adopt elements of primary care for complex patients. Most importantly, they offer ready examples of pragmatic complex care management models.

HIV care models grew out of the discontinuous events of the explosive HIV epidemic in the 1980s. Comprehensive HIV centers care for HIV positive patients with state of the art treatment. Due to the well-known high rates of comorbid psychiatric illness in this population, many such clinics have psychiatrists as well as other mental health personnel and social work on staff. Given the complexity of HIV medications, many also have clinical pharmacists.

Similarly, cancer centers often offer integrated psychiatric and other mental health services in an embedded model of care. Management of delirium and neurocognitive and mood/psychotic disorders caused by cancer and/or cancer interventions can thus be efficiently accomplished with ready access to psychiatric consultants to co-manage cases with oncologists. Treatment in cancer centers may be limited for the duration of active cancer treatment, with patients returning to primary care once cancer management is reduced to surveillance over time.

The models presented here for care of complex cases in structured settings and office-based practice are comprehensive and include components for addressing patients' systemic medical, psychiatric, and social requirements.

There is an additional reality, however. Unfortunately, the resources, time, and personnel required for comprehensive clinical care are often not available in community settings and essentially handicap the PCP delivering the care. Yet, as you will see from the case narratives in the second part of this book, there is a competing factor supporting the value of community care, especially for complex cases. In association with their dedicated medical efforts, office-based PCPs characteristically offer personal involvement and continuity that may not be available in institutional settings. In Chap. 6 we will elaborate on this observation. In it we will argue that the community primary care office may be the best setting for the management of many if not most complex cases encountered in practice.

Reference

1. Frankel S, Bourgeois J, Erdberg P. Comprehensive Care for Complex Patients: the medical-psychiatric coordinating physician model: Cambridge, Cambridge University Press; 2013.
2. Engel G. The need for a new medical model: a challenge for biomedicine. Science. 1977;196:129–36.
3. Bower P, Gilbody S. Stepped care in psychological therapies: access, effectiveness and efficiency. Br J Psychiatry. 2005;186:11–7.
4. Ritchie C, Andersen R, Eng J, et al. Implementation of an Interdisciplinary, Team-Based Complex Care Support Health Care Model at an Academic Medical Center: Impact on Health Care Utilization and Quality of Life. PLoS One. PMID doi: 10.1371/journal.pone.0148096 Feb 12 2016.
5. Wagner E, Davis C, et al. A survey of leading chronic disease management programs: are they consistent with the literature? J Nurs Care Qual. 2002;16(2):67–80.
6. Disease Management Association of America. http://www.dmaa.org.

Chapter 5
Primary Care Practice: The Structures and Methods Associated with Community-Based Primary Practice

Steven A. Frankel and James A. Bourgeois

This chapter reviews the myriad factors that influence the character and quality of community-based primary care and ultimately the care experienced by the patient. To understand the work of the community-based PCPs, all these factors need to be considered.

People with similar needs but who get care from different sources can hardly expect to receive the same level and quality of care. One determinant is the skill and personal qualities of the involved clinicians. A second has to do with the sources of the care received. Even within the same disease category, care settings may differ markedly in the way they are structured and the quality of the care they offer.

Personal Determinants in Clinical Practice, the Contribution of the Clinician and the Patient

Medical decisions are a product of the physician's skill, knowledge, and judgment. Clinical judgment is largely rooted in education, experience, and opinion.

S.A. Frankel, MD (✉)
Department of Psychiatry, University of California, School of Medicine, San Francisco, CA, USA
e-mail: saf@stevenfrankelmd.com

J.A. Bourgeois
Department of Psychiatry, Baylor Scott & White Health, Central Texas Division, Temple, TX, USA

Department of Psychiatry, Texas A and M University Health Sciences Center, College of Medicine, Temple, YX, USA

Department of Psychiatry, University of California San Francisco, School of Medicine, San Francisco, CA, USA
e-mail: James.Bourgeois@BSWHealth.org

© Springer International Publishing AG, part of Springer Nature 2018
S.A. Frankel, J.A. Bourgeois (eds.), *Integrated Care for Complex Patients*,
https://doi.org/10.1007/978-3-319-61214-0_5

"

Clinical Judgment

Physicians make hundreds of decisions during every office visit. These are usually small decisions that microscopically influence the course of treatment. While some such decisions are routine enough to be almost reflexive, many involve significant deliberation requiring disciplined clinical judgment. Involved in clinical judgment are (1) clinician-originated factors that include the clinician's training, experience, medical knowledge, and personal capacity for organizing and prioritizing clinical data and (2) patient-derived factors, which may include examinations and clinical interviews, information from collateral sources such as other professionals and family members, and data from laboratory tests and diagnostic imaging. While the physician generally remains the central figure in clinical decision making and implementation, contemporary medical practices frequently – and often prominently – incorporate additional health-care personnel whose training defines their clinical contributions. Included are licensed practical nurses (LPN), registered nurses (RN), nurse practitioners (NP), physical therapists (PT), occupational therapists (OT), and medical assistants (MA).

It is impossible to remove the human substrate from clinical work, the judgment that goes into all clinical decisions. Subjectivity can enter into clinical judgment through the "clinician-originated" sources described in the previous paragraph (e.g., the clinician's preferences, personal opinions, and predilections) or "patient-derived" sources (e.g., the patient's preferences, opinions, and predilections filtering information communicated to the clinician). It should be clear, then, that clinical judgment exists in partnership with but is often distinct from the technical factors contributing to clinical decision making. "Data" are always commingled with the interpretation and opinion in clinical practice.

Decisions by Physicians: The Implementation of Clinical Judgment

Orchestrating treatment introduces multiple considerations into the clinical process. Beginning with the available data and exercising clinical judgment, the physician, in collaboration with consultants and clinical staff, undertakes a series of actions – major and minor – that together constitute a clinical strategy. Some of these components may be deliberately worked out in the clinician's mind in advance of actions taken. Others may be more spontaneous (but no less complex).

Stanley, a 62-year-old veteran of three spinal surgeries and two psychotherapies, illustrates how judgment enters into the clinical process. Stanley was referred for treatment of his anxiety and pain. Stanley had recently moved and was forced to give up his cherished PCP and local psychiatrist of many years. Stanley was aware that his psychiatric treatment was going to end sooner or later anyway, since his psychiatrist, Dr. L., was being treated for the end-stage complications of multiple sclerosis.

Stanley entered the treatment with his new psychiatrist with barely contained anger. According to Stanley, from the very beginning everything his new psychiatrist did was "wrong." His office was "too hard to find." The picture on his website led Stanley to expect him to be younger, and, to make matters worse, when Stanley missed his second appointment, he was charged for it. That Stanley had never bothered to cancel the appointment apparently did not count. Stanley's argument, after the fact, was that his wife had experienced a "personal emergency" at the time of the appointment, making it hard for him to pay attention to the appointment.

The current psychiatrist decided to "hang in" with the treatment and manage Stanley's confrontations. Of note, however, he was put off by Stanley's attitude and had to struggle personally to keep his irritation from influencing his behavior with Stanley. He managed his reaction in part by personally deconstructing the situation. He hypothesized that Stanley's strident complaints might represent displaced disappointment and anger toward Dr. L. in response to her loss. Since Dr. L. was terminally ill, it seemed likely that Stanley would have difficulty revealing his feelings directly to her or even tolerating them within himself. The current psychiatrist's clinical judgment, his strategy, was based on clinically informed inference. Consequently, in addition to acknowledging and initiating treatment for Stanley's pain, he began to inquire about Stanley's feelings about Dr. L.'s decline and noted that Stanley could be feeling abandoned by her and angry at her for that. As they discussed this issue, Stanley's antagonism began to abate and they were able to progressively refocus on Stanley's pain and anxiety.

Constraints on Practice: Standards of Care: What They Are; How They Are Established

Medical care is not delivered in a vacuum. Getting it right is often a matter of life or death; professional reputation and legal vulnerability may also be relevant but in the background.

Standards of medical care are continually in flux, differing according to illness, circumstance, technology, and evolving practice norms. "Standard of care" specifies appropriate treatment based on scientific evidence (evidence-based care) and collaboration among medical professionals involved in the treatment of a given condition. In legal terms, the applicable standard of care is generally considered care of a quality that a prudent clinician in the relevant specialty and in a given community would provide in a similar case. This standard necessarily reflects how similarly qualified physicians would reasonably manage a patient's care. "Standard of care," is necessarily self-adjusting. Practically speaking, whatever a reasonable primary care clinician would do when presented with a complex case is by definition the standard of care for that case. In a manner of speaking, Stanley, in the last clinical example was questioning his new psychiatrist's standard of care, assuming that he would be receiving substandard care from him.

Standards of care are generally applicable to discrete, definitive diagnoses, such as congestive heart failure or type 2 diabetes mellitus, while complex cases typically have multiple illnesses plus behavioral, social, and/or financial components the requirements of which may conflict or prevent the prudent clinician from precise application of typical standards for treating a single disease entity. The standard of care for complex cases, like Stanley's, is not always as clear as it is in more conventional cases [1].

Common Reimbursement Types for Medical Practices

Practice (care delivery) models, such as multidisciplinary group practices, are structured to generate profits for providers while making care accessible to patients. Efficiently accomplishing this goal requires providers to choose among different reimbursement strategies that best fit their business and clinical goals.

Managed Care

Managed care is most often utilized by organizations and professionals that bear the risk of medical costs for enrollees and seek to minimize those costs. These objectives are sustained while striving to maintain enhanced care quality through a variety of different clinical practice and reimbursement strategies. "Managed care" is a broad term and encompasses many different types of payment mechanisms, review mechanisms, and collaborations within a variety of organizations.

Managed care payers include health maintenance organizations (HMOs), independent practice associations (IPAs), and preferred provider organizations (PPOs). These risk-bearing organizations contract with clinicians who accept risks of enrollee care costs in exchange for a stream of patient business. As discussed earlier, this end is accomplished through different kinds of reimbursement strategies (e.g., capitation, performance bonuses, or cost-limited fee-for-service payments).

As a means to reimbursement, HMO participation can provide incentives to physicians through rewarding care quality and providing cost savings bonuses. Achievement of these goals is judged according to validated metrics. A parallel focus on both quality of care and cost savings is well embedded in health policy development and requires the alignment of economic and clinical incentives. These incentives are not unrelated: improved care quality translates to economic benefits in part through reduced treatment cost. The key to successfully aligning hospitals and physicians is integration between the two areas and joint incentives for academic, quality of care, and clinical productivity.

The Rationale for HMO Type of Care Payment Arrangements: The Traditional Fee-For-Service Model Versus Shared Savings

Private practices and private practice organizations (PPOs) tend to be tied to fee-for-service payments. This means that the provider gets paid more if more medical services are offered. Therefore, there is a financial incentive for providers to perform services (in volume and in kind) that drive-up the overall cost of care. However, this additional cost does not necessarily tie back to improved care quality. Stated differently, the financial interest of the insurer (lower costs) is not aligned with the financial interests of the physician (higher payment). Since the insurer is paying for the services out of a fixed amount of premiums paid by beneficiaries and the insurer's profit depends on utilization over which the insurer does not have control, the insurer is said to be "at risk" economically in this arrangement.

Reconciling the two motivations is the principle of "shared savings." Cost savings is a payment arrangement incentivizing providers to reduce health-care spending for beneficiaries by offering them a percentage of net savings realized as a result of their efforts. For example, if an insurer determines that the cost of care for a defined patient population this year will be $X, and if the actual cost of care for the population (which is generally controlled by physicians) is 80% of that amount, then according to the principle of "cost savings" the insurer may agree to share part of the 20% "savings" with the physicians.

Reconciliation of the Disparate Interests of Practitioner and Economy of Practice

The HMO is an attempt to align the disparate financial interests of providers and the need for economy in practice. HMO participation allows physicians to share in the economic risk of the care provided through negotiated "capitation payments" from the insurer (e.g., the insurer pays the provider a fixed dollar amount to offer all the health-care services of certain types that are needed by a defined group of patients in a given year). As opposed to fee-for-service arrangements, capitation arrangements encourage providers with financial incentives to bring health-care costs down (e.g., if fewer services are provided, more of the capitation payment will be available for provider profit or income). Here, the providers, in theory, have a financial incentive to use more minimal, effective, and preventative care than they do under the fee-for-service model. Additionally, to financially incentivize providers not to just perform minimal services but also to improve care quality, HMOs can offer providers certain kinds of bonus payments for health-care quality outcome measures. Of note, capitation payment arrangements are usually best handled by larger practices that have the sophistication and resources to make the most accurate estimates of actual patient costs.

ACOs

An accountable care organization (ACO) is, in general terms, a set of providers from various organizations who agree to be accountable for the quality and cost of care for a group of beneficiaries. This alignment structure is an innovation designed to produce better care at lower cost for the community. Providers may form an ACO for a number of reasons including (1) coordination of clinical activities involving private third-party payors or (2) to participate in the Medicare Shared Savings Program or other care delivery reforms and associated experiments that are set forth in the Patient Protection and Affordable Care Act (PPACA).

Regulations promulgated under PPACA establish requirements for forming an ACO and require at least a formal legal governance, and management structure, a minimum number of beneficiaries, and certain processes to promote evidence-based medicine and quality/cost analyses. A qualifying ACO may be eligible to contractually agree to be clinically and financially responsible (accountable) for the care of certain assigned fee-for service beneficiaries; e.g., beneficiaries for whom the ACO professionals provide the bulk of primary care services. ACOs that participate in and maintain compliance with the terms of these alternative reimbursement programs (e.g., the Medicare Shared Savings Program) may be eligible to receive shared savings payments and distribute them among their clinicians if certain quality and cost targets are achieved. The accountability requirements for care quality are quite specific and well embedded in the rules governing ACOs (see earlier mention of the "triple aim").

We note that while the new administration in Washington has stated its opposition to PPACA, it is unclear at the time of this writing whether and how it will change (by law or regulation) the ACO rules or the Medicare Shared Savings Program in which PPACA ACOs may participate. While one purpose of PPACA ACOs is to control or limit Medicare expenditures, it is conceivable that the current Administration may favor alternative cost control approaches such as bundled payments, utilization limitations, or simpler price reductions. The health-care regulatory environment is frequently changing, and health-care industry participants will need as always to build in the potential for wide-ranging regulatory shifts in their long-term strategic planning.

Care Delivery, Common Types of Practice

Solo Practice

In most situations, office-based care centers on a treatment team under the supervision of a physician, a physician assistant (PA), and/or a nurse practitioner (NP). Other team members may include Licenced Practical Nurses (LPN), Registered Nurses (RN), a case manager (CM), medical assistants (MA), physical or occupational therapists (PT/OT), and a variety of administrative staff for billing and record keeping.

Multispecialty Group Practice

Most physicians who are located outside a major medical center practice in small multispecialty groups. These practice groups (as opposed to solo practitioners) have the advantage of service diversity, with a variety of specialists available for patient referral and consultation within the same practice. As with any group practice, multispecialty groups vary widely in structure and size. Some are independent, some are affiliated with hospitals or health systems, and still others (in states without a corporate practice of medicine prohibition) are owned and operated by hospitals or health systems. Accordingly, multispecialty group practices vary widely in their governance style, care quality, accesses to external (outside of the multispecialty group) specialists, and ability to service capital needs (such as may be necessary to deploy sophisticated technology). In practice groups associated with larger institutions, while physicians may retain a vote on practice standards, the institution's administration is responsible for most other major practice decisions, strategic initiatives, and/or capital and operating budgets, as well as billing and collections. In physician-owned multispecialty clinics, physicians typically play a more direct role in operational matters and may take turns in leadership roles for the group. A large, physician-owned clinic may appoint a board director to oversee operations, with a professional executive administrator hired to carry out the board's objectives.

Major Medical Center

For practices within the major medical center policies, including allocation of resources, are based on sophisticated medical and financial principles that incorporate the center's academic goals. Major medical centers are typically distinguished by the state-of-the-art care they provide. Once relatively isolated from primary and secondary care medicine and existing mainly as referral destinations for tertiary and quaternary care patients, major medical centers are increasingly competing (through foundations, networks, and other business vehicles) in the primary and secondary care markets in which solo practitioners and multispecialty groups operate.

Who Actually Delivers the Care?

Who are the people actually delivering the care? In each clinical situation how directly is a physician involved in the care of the patients?

In organizations employing various disciplines of health-care professionals, care duties are being increasingly allocated to allied health-care professionals with physicians increasingly shifted to administrative or consultative roles [2]. The following catalogue represents an extensive, yet incomplete typology that includes physicians and allied health-care professionals. The organization of the care, who is employed, to what extent, and for what purpose, differs from setting to setting.

In considering this question, note that the PCP is often also involved with or works in parallel with a number of "shadow supports," health-care-associated professionals or organizations that may enhance or complicate a patient's health-care situation and who are likely to be certified within their own professional organization. Included are organizations like Alcoholics/Narcotics Anonymous, chiropractors, acupuncturists, or individual clinicians who represent themselves as providing partial or full treatment for systemic medical illnesses. This dimension adds complexity to the care situation that may not ordinarily be recognized or acknowledged.

Primary Care Physicians

The backbone of the collective group of medical practitioners is primary care physicians, including family physicians, internists, and pediatricians. Obstetrics and gynecology physicians (ob-gyn) are sometimes included with "primary care."

Physician Assistant

Physician assistants (PAs) may lead a treatment team under the supervision of a physician. The following definition is from the American Academy of Physician Assistants (2014):

> Physician assistants are health professionals licensed or, in the case of those employed by the federal government, credentialed to practice medicine in association with designated collaborating physicians. Physician assistants in the USA are qualified by graduation from an accredited physician assistant educational program and/or certification by the National

> Commission on Certification of Physician Assistants. Within the physician-physician assistant relationship, the physician assistant provides patient-centered medical care services as a member or co-leader of a healthcare team. Physician assistants practice with defined levels of autonomy and exercise independent medical decision making within their scope of practice.

The scope of a PA's practice can vary according to jurisdiction (state or country) and health-care setting. Accordingly, their work may include conducting physical exams, ordering and interpreting tests, diagnosing illnesses, developing treatment plans, performing procedures, prescribing medications, advising on preventive health care, and assisting in surgery [3].

Nurse Practitioners

Nurse practitioners (NP) include advanced practice registered nurses (APRN) who are educated and trained to provide health promotion and maintenance through the diagnosis and treatment of acute illness and chronic conditions. According to the International Council of Nurses, an NP/APRN is "a registered nurse who has acquired the knowledge base, decision-making skills, and clinical competencies for expanded practice beyond that of an RN, the characteristics of which would be determined by the context in which he or she is credentialed to practice" [3]. The main categories of specialization for NPs are adult (ANP), acute care (ACNP), gerontological (GNP), family (FNP), pediatric (PNP), neonatal (NNP), and psychiatric-mental health (PMHNP). Nurse practitioners (NPs) manage acute and chronic medical conditions, both physical and mental, performing history and physical exam and ordering of diagnostic tests and medical treatments with a focus on health-care maintenance. With restrictions that differ from state to state, NPs are qualified to diagnose medical problems, order treatments, perform some advanced procedures, prescribe medications, and make referrals for acute and chronic medical conditions within their scope of practice. NPs work in hospitals, private offices, clinics, and nursing homes/long-term care facilities.

In the United States, depending upon the state in which they work, nurse practitioners may or may not be required to practice under the supervision of a physician. In consideration of the shortage of primary care/internal medicine physicians, many states are eliminating "collaborative practice" agreements so that nurse practitioners are able to function independently [4].

Other Physician Support and Supplement Personnel

Included in this category are health professionals and technicians who may have wide ranging clinical responsibilities and may be assigned to a case by a health-care agency or insurance company. These professionals include care and case managers, care navigators, and health coaches. Care managers and case managers (often nurses or social workers) as well as social workers who provide analogous professional and community liaison services usually have additional training and will be discussed below. In addition to their responsibilities for medical care, they plan interventions to counteract psychosocial and health systems barriers affecting a patient's care.

Care Managers and Case Managers

Care and case managers are adept at planning and orchestrating treatment strategy. Ordinarily there is a physician or other senior clinician who administratively supervises the care or case manager. That person takes ultimate responsibility for approving clinical decisions. The use of case and care managers is growing, in part because of their value for facilitating integrated care as well as the economic advantages associated with their use [5].

The Commission for Case Manager Certification® is the first and largest nationally accredited organization that certifies case managers. It is a nonprofit, volunteer organization that oversees the process of case manager certification. Professional certification is a voluntary process by which a nongovernmental professional organization grants recognition to an individual who has met certain qualifications. The credential attests that the individual has demonstrated a certain level of mastery of a specific body of knowledge and skills within the relevant field of practice. The Case Management Society of America provides analogous certification and sponsors an extensive training program for case managers.

Credentialing organizations for case managers include:

ACHC – Accreditation Commission for Health Care
ANCC – American Nurses Credentialing Center
CARF – Commission on Accreditation of Rehabilitation Facilities
NCQA – National Committee for Quality Assurance
URAC – Utilization Review Accreditation Commission
CMSA – Case Management Society of America

Integrated Case Managers (ICMs)

This is a relatively new designation for care managers who provide medium to high intensity assistance and support for combined systemic medical and psychiatric/mental health treatment for "complex patients." According to Kathol and Cohen (2010) "Complex patients are those with high health complexity and cost (10% to 15% of patients)" [6]. These case managers have advanced training in integrated case management. A current upgrade of Kathol's designations and procedures applicable to integrated case management is called "value-based integrated case management" (VB-ICM). This enhanced version of case management has the objective of bringing additional value to treatment through sophisticated case management as measured by the triple aim of treatment success, patient satisfaction, and economy [5].

Other Health-Care Clinicians and Approaches

The variety of additional health-care practitioners and methods are too numerous to list here. Conventional health-care practitioners not already identified include surgeon's assistants, athletic trainers, midwives, dietitians, marriage and family therapists, psychologists, social workers, occupational therapists, physical therapists, radiotherapists, respiratory therapists, audiologists, speech pathologists, optometrists, dentists, podiatrists, and a wide variety of other clinicians trained to provide some type of health-care service. They often work in hospitals or health-care centers [7].

Approaches to treatment from outside of conventional, evidence-based Western medicine are many. Examples include practices such as homeopathy, naturopathy, chiropractic, energy medicine, various forms of acupuncture, Chinese medicine, Ayurvedic medicine, Sekkotsu, and Christian faith healing [8].

Consumers may have a difficult time choosing among alternative approaches and practitioners, especially when these choices purport to offer simpler or more affordable cures than those that are traditionally considered acceptable. Overall, 34% of adults in the United States used a complementary medicine approach in 2012 [9].

Outcome: The Result of the Shift of the Responsibility from Physicians to Support Personnel on the Culture of Medicine

What motivates primary care physicians to remain passionate about their work? With so many supplementary and complementary health professionals providing care, what is the impact on primary care medicine? In organized medicine, "integrated care" is receiving increased attention with some supporters progressively advocating for a reduction of the physician's role to that of a consultant. Overall, physician leadership tends to be reserved for complex cases [10].

Most primary care physicians chose medicine as a career in order to be central in the treatment process. Paradoxically, while there is markedly increased governmental and organizational advocacy for an increased role for primary care in health delivery, reimbursement trends continue to strongly favor specialist care. This fact, together with the narrowing of the primary care physician's role due to replacement by allied health providers may be contributing to the decline in popularity of primary care medicine among young physicians, thereby exacerbating stresses on the country's primary care system. Medical school graduates are choosing employment and practice models that bring more income and stability over less income and more business risk, as for example would be the case if they were to enter a small community primary practice [11].

As a constructive response – and on an optimistic note – we suggest that a shift in physicians' perspectives may usefully bridge this trend. As the health-care climate changes, physicians could profit by shifting their focus to (1) treating and managing the most difficult patients in their specialty, (2) supervising other health-care professionals, and (3) moving their attention to care for challenging populations, such as those replete with the complex cases we describe in this book. With recommendations such as these in mind, the future for physicians as key, technically elevated, participants in a broader and more collaborative health-care enterprise should be quite promising.

Coordination of Care: How do Health-Care Professionals Work Together and Most Effectively Communicate with Patients?

Adequate communication among clinicians is obviously central to providing optimal health care. That medicine is "fragmented" has become a cliché. Everyone who works with and experiences health care knows it. Everyone experiences it. The "elephant in the room" is that imperfect and fractured communication prevails, while "treatment as usual" continues nonetheless. The bottom line is that in a busy clinical practice, time is always scarce, and the cost of physician time is high. Shifting to streamlined, abbreviated, communication such as email messages saves time and money.

Regarding the form and goals of physician-physician communication, there is a difference between communication typical of a consultation and collaboration. "Collaboration" generally involves repeated contacts with members of a health-care team and ongoing shared ownership of the case. A consultation, typically involves one or two meetings with a specialist for the sake of gaining an opinion.

In office-based primary care group practice, direct conversations among health-care professionals may not be difficult to arrange. But even in these situations, time available for physicians to talk is usually scarce and even physicians in small groups may relate to each other like "ships passing in the night."

To facilitate communication with patients outside of office visits, physicians typically chose email through protected online "portals." While this may be the most efficient choice, it is the least personal method of information sharing. With email as the main vehicle for communication in-person (direct or by telephone) conversations between health-care clinicians have become less frequent, and nuances that enrich communication about clinical matters are likely to be sacrificed.

Written clinical chart notes have been replaced by electronic medical records (EMRs). In spite of its numerous advantages, EMRs have the unwelcomed effect of also limiting face-to-face contact between patients and physicians. For significant periods of each office visit, the physician may be riveted to a computer screen making it difficult for the physician to "get to know" the patient and vice versa [12]. Information conveyed nonverbally and details ordinarily exchanged in face-to-face conversations are often omitted during this process.

Leadership and Team Models

Managing the fragmentation in care delivery is one of the major challenges for primary-care-involved physicians. To a point the organization of care into treatment teams can help address these problems. A discussion of some major team-based treatment models follows.

Collaborative Care

This care delivery innovation was introduced in Chap. 3. "Collaborative care" has come to refer to a system of health-care delivery deliberately designed to provide coordinated care, efficiently and economically. "Integrated care," a close relative of collaborative care, provides many of the same benefits as collaborative care. For integrated care the emphasis, however, is on precise and frequent communication within a treatment team. Collaborative Care targets defined patient populations tracked through a registry, measurement-based practice, and a "treatment to target" guideline. In collaborative care treatment models, primary care clinicians and embedded behavioral health professionals provide evidence-based medication and/ or psychosocial treatments, supported by regular psychiatric case consultation and treatment adjustment for patients who are not improving as expected.

Patient-Centered (Primary Care) Medical Home [11]

The patient-centered medical home (PCMH) as a model of care delivery is of particular contemporary relevance in health care. It is a system within which integrated health care is provided by a health-care provider who is usually a primary care physician. It is intended to provide comprehensive and continuous medical care to patients with the goal of obtaining maximized health outcomes. The objective is to have a centralized setting that facilitates partnerships between individual patients and their personal physicians.

The structure of a PCMH differs from location to location, but the objectives are similar. Principles of patient-centered care were ratified by the American Association of Family Physicians, American Academy of Pediatrics (AAP), American Academy of Family Physicians (AAFP), American College of Physicians (ACP), and American Osteopathic Association (AOA) [13]. The patient-centered medical home consists of a team-based health-care delivery model led by a physician. These personal physicians are responsible for coordination of the patient's care across all health-care systems. The PCMH is intended to provide comprehensive and continuous medical care to patients with the goal of "maximized health outcomes." Care coordination is an essential component of the PCMH and requires resources such as health information technology and appropriately trained staff to provide coordinated care through team-based models. It is noteworthy that the PCMH is a physician-led treatment team concept. While a care or case manager may be essential to the treatment team, the team is led by a physician.

The Medical-Psychiatric Coordinating Physician Model of Care (MPCP)

The Medical-Psychiatric Coordinating Physician model is a physician-led patient care model involving a multispecialty treatment team. It is designed for the treatment of highly complex cases. These cases as we have noted, are both ubiquitous in clinical practices and exceedingly challenging to understand and treat. A "Medical-Psychiatric Coordinating Physician" (MPCP), when embedded in a specialty area, may share team leadership. For example, the MPCP may be a psychiatrist embedded in a medical clinic where administrative leadership is assigned to an internist. Nonetheless, the MPCP has major leadership responsibilities for the cases with which he or she is involved.

As team leader the MPCP has primary responsibility for initiating medical, psychiatric, and surgical work-ups for highly complex cases, maintaining ongoing communication with the patient and often representatives of the patient's family and formally tracking treatment progress. In short, the MPCP is in charge of and fully engaged in the leadership and treatment of these cases. For more responsive (less complex) cases, especially those with significant social issues, many of these functions are typically assigned to case managers. Payment models for the support of an MPCP-led clinical efforts vary according to setting. This new model of care may be especially attractive and appropriate for those physicians who have completed dual training in systemic medicine and psychiatry [14].

Administrator-Led Models

This type of leadership model is ubiquitous in managed care, for-profit hospitals and clinics, and in medical centers where authority over care decisions is hierarchical. This model relies on administrator direction, generally with health-care professionals serving as consultants. Treatments (utilization) are routinely reviewed to assure that resources are used efficiently and according to organizational guidelines. Conflict management is an inevitable part of the administrator's task. For example, conflict may occur between physicians, between physicians and staff, or between the staff of the health-care team and the patient or patient's family. These conflicts may range from disagreements to major controversies involving litigation. These conflicts must be managed vigorously and judiciously to avoid adverse effects on productivity, morale, and patient care.

Concierge Medicine and Other Creative Models

Concierge medicine refers to a relationship between a patient and a primary care physician in which the patient pays an annual fee or retainer generally ranging from $500 to $3000. The objective for this care arrangement is to optimize physician personal responsivity for patient care. In exchange for the retainer, concierge physicians provide enhanced care that includes a commitment to limit their patient caseloads to ensure adequate time and availability for each patient. While all "concierge" medicine practices share similarities, they vary in their structure, payment requirements, and principles of operation. Concierge medicine can be provided by individual physicians, or a similar, albeit less personalized version is available through some multispecialty groups [15].

Additional Considerations

Financial

Paying for health care – Historically medical care in the United States was charged for on a fee-for-service basis. However, few people can pay for medical care out of pocket, and most payment for medical care shifted to private and governmental insurance. Limitations on private insurance care were then determined by insurance companies operating within varying degrees of governmental oversight. Coverage restrictions in this system are multiple and idiosyncratic. Contrasting to the competitive atmosphere for health care in the United States are insurance networks and health systems that are truly organized into "single-payer systems." Single-payer health care is a universal health-care system where a "single payer" fund rather than private insurers pays health-care costs. The "single-payer" aspect of this type of system refers to funding, not delivery. A single-payer fund can be associated with private health-care delivery systems, a public delivery system, or a mix of the two.

"Universal health care" (as one form of single-payer health care) refers to an organized health-care system that provides health-care benefits to all persons in a specified region. Several countries, such as Canada and Germany, provide universal coverage to all of the country's inhabitants. That is, all residents are eligible for basic health-care services. Currently this payment system is not available in the United States. While not as inclusive the PPACA, or similar legislation, can potentially make it possible for increased segments of the population to obtain health insurance.

What Physicians Get Paid and for What?

The resource-based relative value scale (RBRVS) is the system in the United States that was used until recently to determine how much a physician's labor is worth. RBRVS was established in 1992 by the federal government to standardize payments made to clinicians participating in Medicare. In this payment system, a relative value unit (RVU) is assigned to each of the three components that factor into the price paid for a service provided by a physician: physician work, practice expense, and malpractice expense. The payment is determined by multiplying the total value of those three factors by a "conversion factor."

RVUs are updated annually based on recommendations by the American Medical Association and its Specialty Society RVS Update Committee (RUC). The CMS (Centers for Medicare & Medicaid Services) uses these recommendations to determine the values of Current Procedural Terminology (CPT) codes, assigned for treatment and other medical services. Reimbursement to physicians is stringently regulated by insurance companies and governmental payors, with very sizable discounts in physician fees from "reasonable and customary charges." The recently repealed Medicare Sustainable Growth Rate (SGR) formula is a prominent example. Physicians who were already losing considerable income treating Medicare patients were being serially penalized (on a yearly basis) with the objective of correcting huge outflow of money for health care. In response to severely curtailed reimbursement from Medicare, many established physicians have declined to become Medicare participants.

Until recently time spent collaborating with other physicians and family members was not reimbursable by public or private insurance. The 2013 CPT (Current Procedural Terminology) [16] code revisions provided reimbursement for "interactive complexity," a designation involving four specific communication factors that can complicate and prolong care management. Adequate management of complex cases often requires communication/collaboration outside the physician-patient relationship e.g. with health care agencies. While official recognition of these treatment confounders is welcomed, it remains to be seen whether these CPT "complexity codes" will provide adequate support for the collaboration required in most multi-person and otherwise complex treatments.

Overall, the issue of physician/medical group reimbursement is being heavily debated with requirements for personal and group participation in government-funded programs undergoing rapid transformation as ACOs, value-based care, and bundled payments for services move into the forefront. Outcome metrics including those measuring patient satisfaction have progressively found their ways into practice, underpinning the requirements for "value-based care." Good outcomes that are achieved efficiently are the goal, not simply "savings" from cost shifting and restriction of services. The goal is to improve outcomes based on the conviction that in a value-based system, achieving and maintaining good health is inherently less costly than treating poor health [17].

Legal Complexity

As a postscript to this review, the ever present issue of legal regulations applied to clinical practice and the potential for repercussions if they are not carefully followed needs to be acknowledged. These are a "shadow" presence hovering in the background of every clinician's mind, potentially coloring all clinical activities.

In this chapter we have continued with our theme of "clinical complexity." We have focused on the complicated nature of care delivery, as opposed to complex medical-psychiatric-social illness itself. The bottom line is that the overriding challenge for practicing clinicians is facing moment-to-moment treatment choices and addressing them in a medically defensible and affordable way. Our final objective, optimizing patient health, must remain in the forefront of all of our efforts. In the next chapter we will move in the direction of solutions. First there is obvious benefit in the creation of collaborative discussion groups such as ours, at the Center for Medicine, Psychiatry, and Psychology. Second we will propose models for working comprehensively and effectively with clinically complex cases and patients.

References

1. Moffett P, Moore G. The standard of care: legal history and definitions: the bad and good news. West J Emerg Med. 2011;12(1):109–12.
2. Raney LE. Integrating primary care and behavioral health: the role of the psychiatrist in the collaborative care model. Am J Psychiatry. 2015;172(8):721–8.
3. American Academy of Physician Assistants. Current AAPA Policies as of July 2016 Related to the Issue of PA Practice Authority, Responsibility, As of July 2016. [updated July 2016].
4. Fairman JA, Rowe JW, Hassmiller S, Shalala DE. Broadening the scope of nursing practice. N Engl J Med. 2011;364(3):193–6.

5. Kathol R, Knutson KH, Dehnel PJ. Physician's Guide: Understanding and Working With Integrated Case Managers, New York: Springer; 2016.
6. Kathol, R and Cohen, J. The Integrated Case Management Manual: Assisting Complex Patients Regain Physical and Mental Health, New York: Springer; 2010.
7. Frankel SA, Bourgeois JA, Erdberg P. Comprehensive care for complex patients: the medical-psychiatric coordinating physician model. Cambridge: Cambridge University Press; 2013.
8. US Dept. of Health and Human Services. Complementary and alternative medicine products and their regulation by the food and drug administration. [Updated March 2, 2007]
9. Clarke T, Black L. National Center for Health Statistics. National health statistics reports Number 78, February. 2015. Available from: https://www.cdc.gov/nchs/data/nhsr/nhsr078.pdf.
10. Raney LE. Integrated care: working at the interface of primary care and behavioral health. Washington, DC: American Psychiatric Publishing; 2014.
11. Goldman LR, Kumanyika SK, Shah NR. Viewpoint: vital directions from the National Academy of Medicine, October 25, 2016, Putting the health of communities and populations first. JAMA. 2016;316(16):1649–50.
12. Chen L, Boufford J. N Engl J Med 2005; 353:1850–1852.
13. American Academy of Family Physicians, American Academy of Pediatrics, American College of Physicians, American Osteopathic Association, Joint Principles of the Patient Centered Medical Home. [Updated March 2007] Available from http://www.ncqa.org/programs/recognition/practices/patient-centered-medical-home-pcmh. March 2007.
14. Frankel SA, Bourgeois JA, Erdberg P. Comprehensive care for complex patients: the medical-psychiatric coordinating physician model. Cambridge: Cambridge University Press; 2013.
15. Knope S. Concierge medicine: a new system to get the best healthcare. Lanham: Rowman & Littlefield Publishers; 2010.
16. American Medical Association. Chicago: Current Procedural Terminology; 2016.
17. Porter ME. A strategy for health care reform — toward a value-based system. N Engl J Med. 2009;361:109–12.

Chapter 6
Community Care, an Optimal Setting for the Treatment of Complex Cases

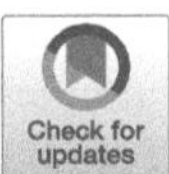

Steven A. Frankel and James A. Bourgeois

Much of medicine is taught in large, highly structured academic medical centers, with access to multiple specialties and subspecialties for treating highly specific, at times esoteric, clinical problems. Physicians who accomplish most of their clinical training in such institutions are accustomed to the access to resources and personnel they provide. As possible, patients with highly complex acute medical/surgical illnesses are preferentially treated at these secondary and tertiary/quaternary care facilities.

In contrast, community-based primary care practice is often more self-contained, the physician typically taking ownership of most manageable cases. The range of readily accessible invasive and other state of the art technically based procedures is more limited than in the academic medical center. However, everything considered, community-based treatment is often the preferred location for chronic complex patients. This treatment model can provide continuity of care over time and the oft-necessary personal-social "engineering" less central to care at the typical academic medical center, where the focus is often on acute management with high-technology and labor-intensive services (e.g., organ transplantation, reconstructive surgery).

S.A. Frankel, MD (✉)
Department of Psychiatry, University of California, School of Medicine, San Francisco, CA, USA
e-mail: saf@stevenfrankelmd.com

J.A. Bourgeois
Department of Psychiatry, Baylor Scott & White Health, Central Texas Division, Temple, TX, USA

Department of Psychiatry, Texas A and M University Health Sciences Center, College of Medicine, Temple, YX, USA

Department of Psychiatry, University of California San Francisco, School of Medicine, San Francisco, CA, USA
e-mail: James.Bourgeois@BSWHealth.org

© Springer International Publishing AG, part of Springer Nature 2018
S.A. Frankel, J.A. Bourgeois (eds.), *Integrated Care for Complex Patients*,
https://doi.org/10.1007/978-3-319-61214-0_6

For the complex patient, what the community-based primary care physician can uniquely offer is an ongoing stable relationship, in which the physician and patient collaboratively address the patient's many difficulties over time. Frequently, complex patients with multiple primary care-level medical problems do not require urgent (as opposed to sustained) attention. Therefore, from early in their treatments, a more longitudinal approach may be preferable for their care. But, even for those who occasionally require secondary or tertiary care, this approach is likely to be effective and in many cases required for the long term. In such a case, the complex patient would be sent from his/her PCP to the academic medical center for evaluation and intervention for a specific medical problem and then returned to the PCP once stable. We will argue that, technical shortcomings of the primary care environment notwithstanding, informed and adequately specialist-supported primary care is the often the better treatment model for highly complex patients.

Is this not a paradox? Should the most complex patients/cases not "deserve" the most technically sophisticated and specialist-intensive care? After all, our current academic medical centers are designed to be prototypes for advanced developments in medical care, where the latest innovations "on behalf of mankind," lofty insights, and epoch-making discoveries are made. Why therefore are they not "the very best" place to take care of the most difficult and often chronically sickest patients (i.e., complex patients and cases)?

To understand this paradox more fully, one must put the illness experience in proper context. Here we use an extreme example. Consider a life saving intervention such as a liver transplant, a dramatic event of life changing proportions. Is this not the proper role for the academic medical center? Should the academic medical center not be the place for the sickest patient, of whatever type.

Yes, but also no. The prototypical orthotopic liver transplant (OLT) patient would likely meet most definitions of "complex patient" based in part on the often encountered comorbid delirium and other psychiatric illness. Added, however, there may be a longstanding history of substance abuse/alcoholism, other systemic medical comorbidities, and the need for recovery programs. Consistently, the bulk of complex patients, and even liver transplant patients, at most points during their clinical course do not have have a major clinical problem that can be reduced to a focal intervention such as an OLT procedure. Most complex patients, as is well known to primary care, have chronic medical illnesses with acute exacerbations and may not need frequent hospitalization based on the course of the main illness. Many complex cases become difficult to manage because of associated clinically distorting psychological and social factors. The academic medical center is not likely to prioritize a focus on the personal, social, and economic needs of patients even if these seriously impede medical treatment and erode the patient's quality of life. Further, continuity of clinic physicians is challenging to accomplish in clinics staffed by residents and faculty members who are responsible for other clinical coverage needs and thus may rotate "off-service" frequently.

Complex patients need a care model that can tolerate their not being "cured" and that focuses on developing means for them to cope with their suffering, as well as accept the inevitability of illness, impairment, and in many cases their demise.

Complex cases typically require "socially engineered" care delivery paired with social interventions, in addition to the medical management of the systemic and psychiatric illnesses that drive their medical presentation. Understanding all of this, the case can be made that *empowered, empathic, and specialty-supported primary care in the community may be the preferred model for care of the typical complex patient.*

A Proposed Model for Primary Care Management of Complex Patients and Cases

A proposed model for the clinical management of medical complexity begins with a committed group of physicians and other professionals who recognize the need for a collaborative model of care. No one can "do it alone." Clinical needs for these patients are almost never encapsulated within a single medical specialty, and even the most committed and skilled generalist (be it a family medicine or internal medicine physician) is unlikely to be current enough with the range of clinical problems to manage a case entirely alone.

However, the keystone to the complex care system is the role of primary care physician. A physician optimally suited to be the primary care physician for complex clinical needs is one with a capacity to "care" as much as "cure" and to accept "process" more than "outcome" in clinical encounters. The dictum that "not all problems can be solved in one encounter" is more true of complex patients than for any others. The physician must be able to empathically connect with the suffering experienced by these patients and be able to understand the patient's other struggles, e.g., in the social aspect of their lives, which often is as unsettling as the pain and suffering caused by the medical syndromes themselves.

The primary care physician for complex patients must be able to appreciate the role of psychiatric comorbidity in important ways. The presence of psychiatric and social comorbidity is part of what makes a "complex" patient "truly complex." The literature is rife with examples of how comorbid psychiatric illness (e.g., major depression) complicates the clinical management of other medical illness (e.g., diabetes mellitus) [1].

For evaluation, the use of psychometric screening instruments (e.g., PHQ-9, GAD-7, MoCA) within the medical care model for both case finding and treatment response monitoring is highly desirable. Added, for the purpose of complexity assessment are (1) a sophisticated assessment tool for clinical complexity called the INTERMED Complexity Assessment Grid (IMCAG) developed by the European-based INTERMED Consortium, and (2) an analogous complexity self-assessment screen, the "INTERMED Self-Assessment" (IMSA) [2].

The primary care physician treating these patients should be able to enter successfully into collaborative treatment relationships with allied health care practitioners as well as with other physicians. Within these treatment relationships, there should be methods of communication between the primary care physician and consultants that include regular meetings to discuss relative progress in cases and outcomes.

Social comorbidity, in contrast, often sets a background "tone" for the case, creating a baseline from which the patient needs to progress. Clearly, an appreciation of the ubiquity of social challenges for complex medical outpatients is essential.

The primary care physician managing complex patients needs access to medical and surgical specialists from specific areas of specialty expertise and specialty-specific invasive procedures, but should remain in overall control of the direction of treatment and outcomes assessment. When the primary care physician refers a complex patient to medical and surgical specialists, he/she should communicate with the consultant about the complexity of the patient, so that the specialist does not view the patient in an overly focal way. Ideally, the primary care physician should have a mechanism to communicate with the involved specialists in order to remain on top of all developments in the patient's treatments.

The primary care physician for complex patients also needs to be comfortable collaborating with allied health professionals who are typically included in the comprehensive care for these complex patients. The list of allied health professionals is long and as elaborated in the last chapter can include among others, nurses and nurse practitioners, psychologists, physician assistants, social workers, occupational and physical therapists, and case managers. Charting needs to be such that clinical communication among the involved professionals is open, reciprocal, pragmatic, timely, and uses common language.

Finally, it is ideal to have regular, structured meetings among the professionals involved in treating complex cases. These meetings should have a collegial and mutually supportive character of course, but can and should also be a forum for detailed and frank discussion about management of complex cases. The treating physicians and other involved professionals can use this regular structured meeting to discuss their experiences, propose directions for management, and use their familiarity with their cases to lend valuable perspectives to the other members of the treatment team.

We propose that when the above elements are available, a community physician-based care model is often the optimum choice for complex patient management. Some benefits to the patient of remaining in his or her geographical community include the greater likelihood of an ongoing relationship with a primary physician and other community-based specialists, regular involvement with assist personnel and services located close to the patient's home, and involvement with nonphysician clinicians who have a connection with and understand the patient's community. These considerations together with the proximity of friends and family members, that is, a personal support system, may lead to the patient feeling personally cared for and result in greater patient motivation to comply with treatment requirements. A relationship with a physician who has been involved with the patient over time may also protect the patient against unnecessary treatments.

Complexity Centers

An idea whose time has come and part of our most ambitious proposal is to recommend the creation of *"complexity centers"* (analogous to cancer centers) wherein a robust clinical model implemented in association with community group multispecialty practices is specifically designed to treat complex patients. Such an institution could establish itself in a given community and seek referrals from other medical clinics, which are less well equipped to provide the comprehensive model of care needed by complex patients. Physicians staffing such centers could be specifically trained to assess, treat, and provide consultation to other health professionals about complex patients and cases.

Consistent with this concept, we conceive of the assessment and treatment of complex patients and complex cases as a *unique area of practice requiring specialized training and experience*. We have previously written about this subject [3] and believe that targeting such populations in this way should have great benefit to the medical community, improving practices and outcomes as well as saving money. We have even visualized clinical complexity as becoming a sub specialization of one of the major medical specialties. A role in comprehensive treatment of complex patients might be especially suited for psychiatrists also trained in internal medicine or family medicine, that is, "dual trained" physicians. Training in combined internal medicine and psychiatry is currently available at 13 medical centers. Another 6 offer combined training in family medicine and psychiatry.

As noted above, we now have available assessment tools, most particularly the INTERMED Complexity Assessment Grid (IMCAG) and its abbreviated version the INTERMED Self Assessment (IMSA) for determining the level and types of clinical complexity. Cases could be screened using these instruments and triaged to the proper types and level of care within the complexity center network.

This concept is in some ways similar to what Roger Kathol has called "Complexity Intervention Units, CIUs." However, according to Kathol, "CIUs, is the suggested new name for what used to be called "Medical Psychiatry Units" (MPUs) or "Psychiatric Medicine Units" (PMUs). Although the clinical activities and personnel working on CIUs will continue to include professionals with public health, mental health, and substance use disorder expertise, changing the name is an attempt to encourage the health system to recognize that the value related to such units occurs most consistently when they are located in general-medical, and not psychiatric, settings and when they target assistance to complex patients, with acute general-medical disorders [4].

As an interesting corollary to our thinking, it might be both practical and forward looking to think of *"clinical complexity" as a diagnostic category in itself*. The complex patient would be referred as a "clinical complexity" case and evaluated using the described screening tools for level and type of complexity. For example, if a patient presented with out-of-control diabetes mellitus with neurological complications, vascular dementia, major depression, alcohol use disorder, and severe personal isolation, the complexity diagnosis would highlight the severity and acuity of each factor, as well as the composite complexity and acuity of the case. In this situation, the assessment might target the diabetes mellitus as needing immediate attention, alcohol dependence as requiring ongoing care including counseling and treatment of major depression as a related measure. The patient's personal situation (e.g., personal isolation) requiring ongoing psychiatric attention might in itself increase the "complexity level" of the case inviting case prioritization in the clinic and the allocation of resources such as psychotherapy, social work, and case management.

As noted in Chap. 5, in 2013, some provisions have been made for payment for collaborative aspects of treatment. "Interactive complexity add-on codes" (referring to CPT add on code 90785) have been appended to the list of CPT codes for covering complicating factors encountered in a patient's visit. "Interactive complexity" is often present with patients who have other individuals responsible for their care including parents, require the involvement of other third parties or schools, and/or need special equipment.

The future: Clearly there is increasing recognition of the public health importance of clinically complex patients. Care delivery structures, job descriptions, and payment methods will need to evolve further for working with this very costly and from a social perspective very problematic segment of the population. We view primary care, optimized to provide appropriate services in collaboration with psychiatry and other mental health professionals, as a distinctly promising direction for these efforts.

References

1. Katon, W, Pedersen, H, Ribe, A. et al. AMA Psychiatry. 2015;72(6):612–619
2. van Reedt Dortland, AKB, Peters, L, Boenink A, et al. Assessment of biopsychosocial complexity and health care needs: measurement properties of the INTERMED self-assessment version (IMSA). Psychosom Med. 2016;79(4):485–492.
3. Frankel, S., Bourgeois, J., et al. (2014) The Medical-Psychiatric Coordinating Physician-Led Model: Team-Based Treatment for Complex Patients. Psychosomatics. 55(4):333–342.
4. Kathol R, Kunkel E, Weiner J, et al. Psychiatrists for medically complex patients: bringing value at the physical health and mental health/substance-use disorder Interface. Psychosomatics. 2009;50(2):93–107.

Chapter 7
Introduction to Case Narratives and Narrative Analysis of Our Collected Cases

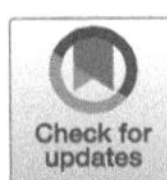

Steven A. Frankel and James A. Bourgeois

Cases can be complicated by an unending array of factors ranging from characteristics of the systems that bound the case, including the family system, the systemic medical and social details of the case, and the personal characteristics of the provider(s) as these affect patient engagement.

In our 16 case narratives, we attempt to illustrate these complexities. They are organized here (1) according to an identifier for the case itself as reflected in the title and (2) a clinical grouping into which the case fits.

Chapter 24 contains an independent narrative analysis of the entire collection of 16 cases. This summary is organized according to the following topics:

1. Provider and health systems factors: including providers' ability to forge an alliance with the patient, provider's ability to manage the patient's systemic medical and psychiatric illnesses, and provider's ability to form alliances with other providers.
2. Patient factors: including the patient's degree of organization, resources, capacity for engagement with providers, and social support.

S.A. Frankel, MD (✉)
Department of Psychiatry, University of California, School of Medicine, San Francisco, CA, USA
e-mail: saf@stevenfrankelmd.com

J.A. Bourgeois
Department of Psychiatry, Baylor Scott & White Health, Central Texas Division, Temple, TX, USA

Department of Psychiatry, Texas A and M University Health Sciences Center, College of Medicine, Temple, YX, USA

Department of Psychiatry, University of California San Francisco, School of Medicine, San Francisco, CA, USA
e-mail: James.Bourgeois@BSWHealth.org

Further order can be achieved by recognizing that major categories constituting clinical complexity can be additionally organized according to (a) patients' systemic medical and psychiatric conditions, (b) social problems, and (c) the dysfunctions and incompatibilities of the health systems where the patient receives services.

The take-home message is the same for all these cases. These cases are organized around complex patients who have multiple illnesses or dysfunctions. Each patient has his or her own subjective experience of illness. Each case requires a creative approach to understanding and management.

What follows is an index for our case narratives. Each full case narrative is prefaced by a summary paragraph and concluded by several paragraphs summarizing the "complexity characteristics" of the case. These complexity characteristics include systemic medical/psychiatric diagnoses (acute and chronic), social considerations (including family and other support systems), care delivery experience, and fundamental factors supporting or obstructing the treatment with special attention to the quality and continuity of the physician–patient relationship. Concluding the book will be a chapter (Chapter 25) summarizing lessons learned from this project.

The titles and authors of these case narratives, arranged according to medical specialty, are as follows:

List of Case Narratives (Arranged by Medical Specialty)

PEDIATRICS
-Steven Frankel, MD, Child and Adult Psychiatry, and Jan Maisel, MD, PhD, Pediatrician

Detailed narrative tracing the development of a major substance use disorder from a patient's birth through his early twenties.

-Steven Frankel, MD, Child and Adult Psychiatry, written with the Patient's Treating Pediatrician Treatment of a case that began as panhypopituitarism, pseudotumor cerebri, but proved to be Munchausen's (factitious disorder) by proxy.

-Steven Frankel, MD, Child and Adult Psychiatry, and Jan Maisel, MD, PhD, Pediatrician

The conflicted treatment of a boy with poor academic and social development and eventual deterioration into psychosis: a pediatrician's struggle to prevail in a hostile treatment environment.

NEUROLOGY
-J. Richard Mendius, MD, Neurologist
A case of parental enmeshment: Two adolescent brothers who initially suffered from a post viral encephalitis accompanied by balance, concentration, memory, and fine motor impairments. Over time, systemic medical indicators were only mildly supportive. The similarity between the symptoms experienced by both boys underscored the probability of an ongoing psychological etiology, consisting of parental encouragement and enmeshment.

-J. Richard Mendius, MD, Neurologist
Longitudinal treatment of a now adolescent boy with history of allergic sensitivity and anaphylaxis as an infant, crippling parental overprotection impeding his social development during childhood, and unconfirmed but claimed epilepsy impeding his social development during his teen years.

FAMILY MEDICINE
– Elizabeth Etemad, MD, Family Medicine
Several-year treatment of Molly, a female with anorexia nervosa (AN), from age 14 to young womanhood. Despite the desirability of psychiatric management of this case, the patient's family refused recommended psychiatric consultation and comanagement, leaving the pediatrician to manage the case. Dr. Etemad describes how she managed this dilemma, providing a psychotherapeutic level of care in addition to medical management of the many medical complications of AN.

– Elizabeth Etemad, MD, Family Medicine
A 68-year-old man whose downhill post-CVA course was complicated by loss of wife's support after she was diagnosed with brain cancer.

COMBINED FAMILY MEDICINE AND PSYCHIATRY
Alvin Lau, MD, Family Medicine-Psychiatry from a County Federally Qualified Health Center (FQHC) Case of complex regional pain syndrome (CARPS) and progressive medical and psychiatric deterioration complex regional pain syndrome with treatment compromised by health systems failures.

PSYCHIATRY
– Paul Gilbert, MD, Psychiatry
A convoluted treatment odyssey involving treatment of severely drug-addicted bipolar woman in her early 20s. Family cooperation critical to case success.

– Paul Gilbert, MD, Psychiatry
A convoluted treatment odyssey involving treatment of severely drug-addicted bipolar woman in her early 20s. Family cooperation critical to case success.

END OF LIFE (INTERNAL MEDICINE)
Curtis (Kip) Roebken, Internal Medicine
End-of-life management where there is family opposition to physician recommended medical measures.

GERIATRIC MEDICINE
– Catharine Clark-Sayles, MD, Geriatric Internal Medicine
Case of escalating interrelated systemic medical and psychiatric illnesses and persistent suicidality.

NEUROLOGY AND INTERNAL MEDICINE
David Palistrant, MD, Neurological Interventionist, Internal Medicine

Case of severe anorexia nervosa requiring hospitalization and parenteral feeding, leading to a legal challenge involving conflict between primary care physician and hospitalists.

SLEEP MEDICINE
Mehrdad Razavi MD, Sleep Medicine and Neurology
47-year-old man with grandiose ideas who refused most medical treatment (other than CPAP) for sleep apnea and eventually took his life.

PAIN MEDICINE
Deepak Sreedharan, MD, Pain Medicine
"Developmental" case with emphasis on treatment of pain and addiction to opioids.

Pain management progressing to addiction to opioids with a 17-year-old boy rendered quadriplegic and by a motorized vehicle accident.

END OF LIFE PLANNING AND MANAGEMENT
Lael Duncan, Internal Medicine, Medical Director of Consulting Services for the Coalition for Compassionate Care of California

This report describes requirements of advanced care planning while anticipating end of life. Two case reports are presented: one a longitudinal presentation of the medical developments in the last decade of a patient's life, and the second describes a woman who fails to comply with planning requirements because of anxiety about abandoning her impaired adult daughter.

Part II
Case Narratives

Chapter 8
Longitudinal Treatment of a Case of Panhypopituitarism, Pseudotumor Cerebri, and (Ultimately) Factitious (Munchhausen's) Disorder by Proxy

Steven A. Frankel

The patient, Eddie, was born by cesarean section at 37 weeks. Eddie was diagnosed with panhypopituitarism by an endocrinologist at age 3 after a significant fall-off in his growth curve. He was started on cortisone, thyroid, and growth hormone replacement with good response.

The fast pacing of the clinical events in this case no doubt reflects the patient's mother's anxiety, her need to see her child as sick, and her complicity in creating clinical urgencies. Dates have been modified or deleted to protect the identity of the patient and his family. The chronology of his complicated systemic medical–psychiatric treatments is as follows (Dates have been modified or deleted to protect the identity of the patient and his family):

- At age 6 years 9 months, Eddie was treated by a pediatric neurologist for episodic headaches and vomiting sometimes accompanied by auras, which were diagnosed as classic migraine. Initially, he was medicated with butalbital, acetaminophen, and caffeine.
- At age 8 years 6 months, Eddie experienced increased, near-daily, headaches with associated vomiting. He was then was treated with levetiracetam, initially with good response.

During this period, there were a flood of medical complaints from both the patient and his mother, resulting in further treatments and specialist referrals. Generally, new problems arose when others improved, and new treatments and consultants were typically added after each incident. The insistence on medical treatment by the patient and his mother was generally pressing, with physicians feeling compelled to attempt whatever standard medical treatments might be available.

S.A. Frankel, MD (✉)
Department of Psychiatry, University of California, School of Medicine, San Francisco, CA, USA
e-mail: saf@stevenfrankelmd.com

© Springer International Publishing AG, part of Springer Nature 2018
S.A. Frankel, J.A. Bourgeois (eds.), *Integrated Care for Complex Patients*,
https://doi.org/10.1007/978-3-319-61214-0_8

Opioids inevitably became re-involved because of Eddie's constant complaints of pain. Some of the events during this period include the following:

- At age 9 years 8 months, when his headaches increased in frequency and severity, levetiracetam was again tried, but without success.
- At age 9 years 9 months, he was admitted to an academic medical center for evaluation. Ophthalmological evaluation revealed papilledema with grossly normal visual fields, pupillary function, and visualacuity. Initial lumbar puncture opening pressure was 32 mm of H_2O (normal 10–20). MRI was consistent with evidence of increased intracranial pressure. He was treated with acetazolamide and four serial lumbar punctures. Significant head and stomach pain were noted throughout his hospital stay, requiring hydromorphone PCA. He was diagnosed with pseudotumor cerebri, presumably secondary to growth hormone treatment which was then discontinued.
- At 9 years 9 months, he was re-admitted for vetriculoperitoneal (VP) shunt placement after failing medical management and acetazolamide was tapered. The summary notes from this admission included, "… he continued to have escalating pain complaints, giving pain numbers of 10/10 and getting escalating narcotic dosing. It became clear that he could be distracted out of much of his pain and that anxiety played a significant component. Child specialists were involved and critical in helping with behavioral and distraction methods. He seemed to respond well to guided imagery." The psychiatric consultant felt that most of what Eddie was calling pain was the result of depression and anxiety, and that he had difficulty distinguishing between psychological and physiological pain. He agreed that Eddie might still be having some pain related to intracranial pressure and headache, but that most of his difficulties were psychiatric." The consultant continued, "The patient and family bring many social stressors to this hospital stay, including a recent divorce, chronic illness and recent surgery for patient's mother, the new diagnosis of autism for his sibling, and diagnosis of cancer for the mother's boyfriend. IN ADDITION THE PATIENT APPEARS TO HAVE BEEN SUPPORTED IN THE ROLE OF THE SICK CHILD FOR MOST OF HIS LIFE AND TO HAVE ESCALATED THAT ROLE SOMEWHAT IN THIS TIME PERIOD WHEN OTHER FAMILY STRESSORS HAVE OCCURRED." (capitalization in the original).

The consultant felt that the patient's mother "appeared to have good insight into these issues, and was quite interested in his continuing therapy as an outpatient." He was started on citalopram 5 mg and amitriptyline 5 mg daily, along with behavioral modalities and (for the time being) was able to wean IV opioids.

When seen a month later by a neurologist, it was noted that, "the patient always has a headache; there is no time of day when he does not have a headache." "He is now sleeping through the night, although he does wake in the middle of the night to move into his mother's bed." The physical exam at that time was normal except for very slight right papilledema. Amitriptyline dose was increased to 10 mg daily.

According to neurology follow-up 4 months later, age 9 years 11 months, "Eddie continues to have daily headache with increased pain and vomiting several times/

week despite trials of PO opioids. He had a 8.3 kg weight gain over prior 3 months. He is missing school two days/week; has no physical education or social activities. Neurological exam revealed allodynia of head/neck areas. Referred for evaluation to a pain clinic and to outpatient psychiatry."

The psychiatry note at that time read, "I feel that in order to adequately treat this child, we need a much more multidisciplinary approach involving consultation by a pain specialist, as well as close involvement by a child psychiatrist and a multidisciplinary team focusing on at both the patient and his family." The psychiatrist concluded, "Reactive depression is now more prominent than anxiety."

- At 10 years 5 months, neurology follow-up note revealed: "No clinical improvement whatsoever despite aggressive medical and psychiatric therapy. There are daily headaches with vomiting and photophobia which increases with stress or fatigue. Attending school less than 50% of the time; often going to work with Mom (who works in clinic for chronic pelvic pain!) resting in a back room. The patient's mother is managing the patient's headaches with prescribed ondansetron, oxycodone, diphenhydramine, acetaminophen, and relaxation techniques."

Shortly afterward, an attempt by the psychiatrist to discontinue amitriptyline because of urinary retention resulted in an "almost immediate severe anxiety reaction, including claimed visual hallucinations, extreme abdominal pain, and emesis." Concern was expressed that "medical management is failing this child."

- At age 10 y 11 m, evaluations at California Pacific Institute for Health and Healing resulted in a recommendation that included acupuncture, craniosacral massage, hypnosis, and guided imagery. Also Eddie's endocrinologist referred him to a university medical center pulmonary clinic to rule out sleep apnea (the patient was overweight and had developed daytime sleepiness). The findings were negative.
- Six months later, at 11 years 5 months, Eddie was weaned off oxycodone by a pain management specialist at a major medical center. He was still having daily headaches, but remained on rizatriptan and gabapentin.
- 11 years 9 months, four months later, Eddie wrote his mother a note stating, "I want to kill myself because I'm fat." The psychiatrist added duloxetine to medication regimen and an insurance supported weight loss program was started.
- 11 years 11 months, two months later, Eddie's family was in a car accident. Mother reported that she sustained "postconcussive syndrome with memory changes, depression, and inability to work."
- Three months later, at age 13 years 4 months, Eddie was admitted to another academic medical center for intensive pain and psychiatric management. Methadone was successfully weaned and he tolerated oral feedings.
- At age 13 years 4 months, Eddie was re-admitted to an academic medical center for 3 weeks for recurrent vomiting and abdominal pain. Upper GI series and an abdominal computerized tomography (CT) scan were normal. Endoscopy revealed mild inflammation of his gastric antrum but all biopsies were normal. He was given bowel rest and TPN for 2 weeks. Three months later, Eddie was again re-admitted to an academic medical center with fever and feeding intolerance.

Blood culture from a peripherally inserted centeral catheter (PICC) line was positive for Serratia Marcescens. He remained hospitalized for the next 3 months manifesting multiple problems related to gastrojejunal tube difficulties, feeding, chronic pain, opioid dependence and psychiatric symptoms. The GI service ultimately decided that Eddie had no primary GI motility problem. Current symptoms were likely due to opioids. A child protrective service (CPS) referral for Munchausen syndome by proxy was considered, but not acted upon due to a disagreement between attending physicians at the medical center. Eddie remained on IV methadone and morphine PCA. Eddie was re-admitted to the same medical center for gastrojejunal tube placement. He was re-admitted 24 h later for feeding intolerance.

– During this period, the mother became capricious, refusing care from doctors with whom she disagreed. She felt a gastrojejunal tube should have been inserted. After prolonged discussion, it was agreed that a gastric-emptying study should be repeated, at 13 years 4 months. The repeated study was markedly abnormal (he was off opioids for the study). He was diagnosed with "gastroparasis of unknown etiology."

At 13 years 5 months, Eddie was again readmitted and remained for 3 months. During this second admission, there were multiple problems with the feeding. Eddie's motility problems were ultimately attributed by the GI service to opioids.

At this point, 14 years 0 months, Eddie's mother separated from her husband (who entered an inpatient alcohol rehabilitation program). The mother had taken up residence in patient's room. His younger brother spent the school vacation in that room as well. Within weeks Eddie was transferred to a university medical center, for intensive pain and psychiatric management. He was discharged 4 months later.

– Days later, Child Protective Services (CPS) was contacted by a medical center social worker. Several days later, the patient and his younger brother were removed from their mother's care and transferred to their father's house. Court proceedings alleging that the mother was causing the patient to undergo unnecessary medical procedures resulted in the mother losing legal and physical custody, with all visitations supervised and no feeding of any kind by her allowed. Subsequently, there was a return office visit with Eddie accompanied by his father. "Eddie's weight was 150 pounds and he was "doing very well – no vomiting." He had entered the eighth grade at a new school and was getting "As." Nonetheless, Eddie still claimed that he "always" had a headache.

– There were no office visits for over 1 year. Eddie was brought in for a complete physical exam at age 14 years 2 months. At that point, Eddie was in high school and getting straight As. Weight 169 pounds height 65.5 "with BMI 27.7 kg/M2, He had some pubic hair but testes and penis were still prepubertal. He was still prohibited from school sports and physical education by the medical center physicians due to the VP shunt, but the father was working on increasing exercise at home. There was no mention of any pain during entire visit. The father reported that Eddie was having no apparent pain or other physical or emotional problems at home. According to his pediatrician, he now seemed able to tolerate and get through illness "like a normal kid."

Case Summary

From early in his life this patient's course was complex, with systemic medical illness regularly eclipsing psychiatric comorbidity in the opinions of his consulting physicians. There were two other potent sources of distortion contributing to the always evolving complexity of the case. The first was the consulting physicians' preference for (and greater familiarity with) systemic medical explanations for the patient's presentations. Their overweighting of the these issues appears to have resulted in underestimation of the psychological underpinnings of the patient's medical presentations. The second, and more important influence, was the mother's almost fanatical insistence that her son was vulnerable and sick. Eddie's broad-minded, community based pediatrician, however, was able to maintain a balanced view of his illnesses throughout the case and guide the case through its multiple vicissitudes.

Complexity Summary

1. Biological (including genetic)
   Acute:
   - Principle diagnosis: elevated intracranial pressure/pseudotumor cerebri (with shunt)
   - Secondary diagnosis: panhypopituitarism
   Chronic:
   - Munchausen's syndrome by proxy (complicit insistence that the patient had intensive medical requirements by mother and child)
2. Psychiatric/psychological
   - The patient's hyperreactivity to pain and reported allodynia. These developments were apparently significantly facilitated by the mother's own anxiety and excessive attachment needs.
   - Patient's coexisting anxiety disorder and depressive disorder, diagnosed and treated.
3. Social stressors (including family and other support systems)
   - Strained relationship between parents leading to their separation at patient's age 14.
   - The patient's social relationships were delayed, presumably reflecting his having been indulged and sequestered by mother.
4. Care delivery, including access to care
   - There was a generous supply of medical resources available, with probable overuse of these.
5. Fundamental factors supporting or obstructing the treatment, in particular the quality and continuity of the physician—patient relationships
   - The mother's complicity with the patient's claimed suffering gave consulting physicians little choice other than to treat symptoms. Paradoxically, these treat-

ments may have assisted mother and child in maintaining child's compromised state by focusing unrelenting attention on his medical symptoms.
– This case raises the question of when a physician (the consulting physicians in this case) should decide "I can't manage the case." Maintenance of medical treatment by multiple skilled consulting physicians through patient's age 14, while in compliance with a high standard of medical practice, ironically may have contributed to perpetuating the essential problem which we infer was the mother's need to have a sick child.

Chapter 9
A Boy with Poor Psychosocial Development and Eventual Psychotic Disorder: A Pediatrician's Struggle to Prevail in a Hostile Treatment Environment

Steven A. Frankel and Jan Maisel

This is a complex pediatric case, followed from age 8 to adulthood. The patient initially presented with allergic-spectrum illness complicated by poor social and academic performance. A major disruptive issue from the start of treatment was profound disagreement between the (divorced) parents about managing their son's healthcare. The result of this breach was disruptions of care adherence and thus, continuity. Legal involvement was ultimately necessary to manage this case. The patient's psychiatric illness was itself complex (including elements of anxiety, depression, and psychosis) and created increased challenges in care for an already highly complex case.

It begins with the diagnosis of severe allergies, the external manifestations of which (eczema, wheezing, red eyes, dry skin, and unremitting exhaustion) created the impression of a "very miserable child." Laboratory studies were consistent with an atopic (asthma and allergic rhinitis) etiology. Oscar also had significant tonsillar hypertrophy. Spirometry was mildly abnormal but responsive to bronchodilators. Medications included an inhaled corticosteroid, albuterol MDI (metered dose inhaler), montelukast, cromolyn, pimecrolimus, and prescription and over-the-counter steroid creams. Dust control measures were implemented. Over the next few years, there was a gradual improvement in asthma control (from "moderate persistent" to "mild intermittent") but with persistent nasal, eye, and skin symptoms essentially year-round.

S.A. Frankel, MD (✉)
Department of Psychiatry, University of California, School of Medicine, San Francisco, CA, USA
e-mail: saf@stevenfrankelmd.com

J. Maisel, MD, PhD (✉)
University of California, Medical Center, San Mateo, CA, USA

Tamalpais Pediatrics, Larkspur, CA, USA
e-mail: janmaisel@gmail.com

© Springer International Publishing AG, part of Springer Nature 2018
S.A. Frankel, J.A. Bourgeois (eds.), *Integrated Care for Complex Patients*,
https://doi.org/10.1007/978-3-319-61214-0_9

Oscar had two older siblings. His parents divorced when he was 5 years old. His mother remarried when he was 7 years old. Oscar and his siblings spent every other weekend and a weekday night with his father. His father worked in retail. His mother was a school administrator. Importantly, Oscar's father was preoccupied with the use of nutritional supplements and resistant to conventional treatments. His mother was relatively tolerant of the father's bias, but at the same time was consistently accepting of conventional medicine for Oscar's care.

Strikingly, in spite of his superior intelligence and despite extra academic support introduced in a timely fashion, from early elementary grades, Oscar struggled with academics. His initial school difficulties involved "visual processing" problems and poor graphomotor skills. He also had little interest in or success with peer relations. A psychometric assessment at 7 years of age by the school system revealed superior intelligence (overall IQ 128) but significantly delayed reading and writing skills. He was also assessed as being cognitively and emotionally "at risk." He was cooperative during psychometric testing but generally appeared "exhausted" to the assessing psychologist. The BASC-2 (*Behavior Assessment System for Children, Second Edition*) assessment completed by Oscar's parents and teachers was clinically significant for anxiety, depression, and somatization. Recommendations included daily "pull-out" from class for emotional support and remedial education. His school and social failures continued without reprieve year after year, despite repeated special education remediation.

Oscar returned for an appointment at 9 years of age with complaints of morning stomach aches and fatigue paired with nighttime snoring. Laboratory studies included negative CBC, thyroid panel, celiac panel, and stool H. pylori. Physical exam revealed markedly hypertrophic tonsils, and his pediatrician was concerned about possible sleep apnea as an exacerbating factor in his fatigue and school struggles. Tonsillectomy and adenoidectomy (T and A) were recommended, and an ENT referral was made but was postponed by the mother after consultation with a family member who was described as a "retired nutritionist." Instead, a gluten free-diet was started, despite negative celiac tests.

When the patient was 10 years old, a school-based psychotherapist became concerned about possible physical or sexual abuse and dietary coercion involving nutritional supplements at his father's house. She contacted Child Protective Services (CPS). Oscar and his siblings were interviewed by CPS and a police detective. In the CPS interview, Oscar stated that he always had "a horrible time" at his dad's house. To his pediatrician, he said his dad "massaged" him during each visit in the evening. He stated that areas massaged were upper thighs, and bottom of feet and shoulders. He found this unpleasant and painful. When asked about duration of pain, he replied, "two days for shoulder pain, two hours for thigh pain and fifty minutes for foot pain." When asked if he had told his father that he disliked the massage, he replied "yes, but my father thinks I love it." Oscar denied any massaging of the genital areas. When the pediatrician asked Oscar if there were any fun activities at Dad's, he answered, "His idea of fun is to go to an photo exhibit and stare at a picture for one hour."

Mother stated that the father believed that his children were "wheat and dairy allergic and also lactose intolerant" and was requesting a full nutritional workup. The pediatrician spoke with the father by phone and attempted unsuccessfully to reassure him that there was no medical evidence for wheat or dairy allergy, or lactose intolerance, an opinion shared by the allergist. Child Protective Services ultimately spoke with the father instructing him to refrain from massages and to discontinue insisting on nutritional supplements for the boys. In response to the CPS intervention, all five family members were referred for family psychotherapy with a social worker.

Soon after this incident, at age 11, Oscar began seeing another psychotherapist, a psychologist, for weekly psychotherapy. The psychotherapist initially made the observation that "Oscar doesn't look well." However, he did not contact the pediatrician, and instead attempted to initiate an extensive and, in the opinion of his pediatrician, inappropriate nutritional workup. The pediatrician reassured the mother that Oscar had no clinical evidence of malabsorption or vitamin deficiencies, and that both his height and weight were within normal limits, both showing significant interval improvement over the previous year.

Nevertheless, laboratory studies were ordered by a "naturopath" (a nonphysician who specializes in "holistic approaches" to diseases or disorders, who had a relationship with the father. That testing revealed a low vitamin D level and in vitro reactivity to gluten-type proteins, a result that does not correlate well with actual gluten sensitivity. The patient's mother reported that Oscar's nutritional regimen at that time included vitamin D, a magnesium/calcium supplement, aloe vera juice, and a "probiotic." According to the pediatrician, despite this regimen, the psychotherapist continued to express concerns about Oscar's "unhealthy appearance" and kept recommending new workups and supplements. During this period, he never contacted the pediatrician to discuss his concerns or obtain input, whereas Oscar's mother dutifully conveyed the psychologist's suggestions to the pediatrician. At one point, the mother even implemented a 4-week dairy elimination diet and took daily pictures of the patient hoping to demonstrate to the patient's father that the elimination of dairy made no health difference for Oscar.

In response to the CPS incident and the patient's ongoing problems, all family members (patient, parents, and patient's siblings) participated in family psychotherapy with a social work intern. However, Oscar's emotional adjustment continued to deteriorate. At age 12, he began to experience sleep disturbances with nightmares about his mother or himself being killed. At an office visit, he reported a frightening visual images of a "strange man" who was shooting at him. That these experiences seemed real to Oscar suggested that they might be hallucinations, a harbinger of a psychotic disorder. In addition, Oscar was continuing to struggle academically despite a one hour/day resource class and occupational therapy. Because of the apparent lack of progress from the current psychotherapy coupled with onset of probable hallucinations, his pediatrician strongly recommended a child/adolescent psychiatry consultation.

Shortly thereafter, a child/adolescent psychiatrist evaluated Oscar and recommended that treatment be initiated with a trial of an antidepressant, but the father refused permission. Subsequent academic and psychological tests were obtained. The results revealed below average academic scores, yet the school, very oddly, did not diagnose a "learning disorder" in spite of a total reading score in the 9th percentile. Depression and anxiety, resulting in "difficulty with emotional regulation and mood control, as well as poor coping skills," were identified as being of central importance diagnostically. A "emotional disturbance," rather than cognitive or other neuropsychological impairment, was seen as the primary disabling condition.

Oscar's mother soon returned to court with the aim of decreasing overnight stays at the father's home. She felt that Oscar was losing 2 days per week of effective learning due to the stress of each visit with father. She did not have full custody for medical matters but the court had previously mandated that the father must support prescribed conventional medications and could not substitute nonconventional medication not approved by the pediatrician.

When seen again at 14 years old, Oscar had been able to discontinue one of his asthma medications. But his rhinitis was poorly controlled due to his refusal of nasal steroid therapy. Also, his eczema had worsened. His tonsils were still hypertrophic, and he had diffusely dry skin with periorbital erythema, indicative of persistent atopic dermatitis. He was continuing to do poorly personally and academically. Suicidal ideation had been noted along with deteriorating school behavior and performance. A consultation with a new child/adolescent psychiatrist resulted in the presumptive diagnosis of depression and the prescription of an antidepressant (venlafaxine).

Meanwhile, Oscar's psychologist continued to suggest a complementary medicine approach, emphasizing nutrition for his treatment. He also recommended referral to a rheumatologist. In disagreement, his pediatrician recommended a second opinion by an allergist, a choice supported by the mother. Laboratory testing confirmed allergy as the major issue. The mother's position prevailed, and Oscar's medications were adjusted. In addition, his dermatologist instituted measures to better control his eczema because Oscar had developed bacterial folliculitis secondary to its persistence.

The mother's legal case against the father progressed, and by May of that school year, the court granted the mother sole authority to make decisions for medical, educational, and psychological matters. By that time, however, at age 15, Oscar was again articulating suicidal thoughts. At his next annual checkup with his pediatrician he stated: "I don't have the energy to walk up the stairs …I'd rather die than go to school." None of his academic goals had been met. His emotional deterioration continued. During the final 2 months of the school year, he became intermittently assaultive toward his mother. Medically, there were signs of increased stability. His asthma continued to improve, and his inhaled steroid had been discontinued. His tonsils were now normal in size, and his eczema was less problematic. However, a new major medical issue was identified: advanced thoracic scoliosis.

At age 16, an independent and in-depth neuropsychological report was obtained. It read, "The best psychiatric diagnosis at present is major depression with psychotic features." The recommendation was for residential treatment. This recommendation was not supported by the school system, whose financial support would have been necessary for its implementation. In spite of this recommendation, Oscar was forced to enter a public middle school.

Soon after the beginning of the school year, the patient's mother reported to the pediatrician that a week previously Oscar had locked himself in the school nurse's bathroom. When he emerged, he had ripped his clothes and detached some of the brackets supporting his braces. This incident was followed by one in which Oscar attempted to hide a large knife on his body. When his mother took possession of the knife, Oscar collapsed on the floor screaming. This incident was followed by involuntary psychiatric hospitalization for 5 days, where delusional thinking was noted. Following this hospitalization, Oscar's mother argued that her son's deterioration was alarming, and that he required the structure of a facility specializing in the treatment of severely disturbed adolescents. She and Oscar's pediatrician had argued vociferously that the public education system was inadequate and inappropriate for his care. The struggle with the public school system to garner such support had been dramatic and repeatedly discouraging. It was only when Oscar became overtly delusional and suicidal that they relented likely at least partially due to the attorney Oscar's mother ultimately was compelled to retain.

Placement was arranged at a residential psychiatric treatment program for adolescents in a distant state. Several months later, in a phone conversation with the pediatrician, the mother reported, "For the first time Oscar is making a slow crawl to progress in all areas." It had taken 6 weeks for him to begin to integrate into the academic program and for him to stop insisting on going home. His mother was allowed to speak by telephone with him once a week and visit on the extremely limited schedule set by the residential treatment center. Contacts with his father were barred by the court. Gradually, Oscar's anxiety began to ameliorate, and delusional thinking began to disappear. Reportedly, he was beginning to "find some joy in his life."

At age 17, some months later, Oscar went home for a visit. His mother stated, "He is finally successfully doing some academics and has made a few friends." He was off asthma medications. He was taking only topical medication for allergic rhinitis and eczema (which overall had improved). He was also taking duloxetine 60 mg/day for anxiety and depression. There was no remaining evidence of psychotic thinking or suicidal ideation. His PHQ-9 depression index score was now much improved to 8, consistent with mild depression.

At age 18, orthopedic follow-up for Oscar's scoliosis revealed severe progression with a 58 degree curve, making surgical stabilization mandatory. When Oscar's father was informed about the planned surgery, he telephoned Oscar's residential program asserting that Oscar's scoliosis (which was congenital) was "Oscar's own fault" adding, "we store our tension in our spine and if Oscar had done a better job in therapy that would not have happened." He also stated that what Oscar needed rather than surgery was to "hang from the monkey bars and see a chiropractor." He proposed to send Oscar a bar that could be installed in the doorway of his room. The director refused stating that its presence would present a "serious risk in this (therapeutic) school setting." At age 18, Oscar underwent a successful spinal fusion of vertebrae T10-L4. His post-operative recovery was uneventful, without recurrence of any of his psychiatric symptoms, and he continued to progress toward both physical and mental health.

Pediatrician's Reflections

Looking back over my 9 years of involvement with Oscar and his family, the "arc" is that of several relatively severe allergic conditions improving slowly over time, accompanied by learning struggles and depressive, anxiety, and, ultimately, psychotic disorders which gradually moved to the forefront and ultimately became disabling.

I was initially concerned that the onset of Oscar's emotional difficulties could have been triggered by his allergy struggles. I am certain these caused Oscar to never feel like a "healthy kid." I worried that I might have had some responsibility for this progression since I could not prescribe a "magic bullet" that would fully eradicate his allergic symptoms. But the coexisting family issues on top of Oscar's intrinsic emotional vulnerability could just as easily have been the triggering factors. In the end, I was able to let go of my personal sense of responsibility, given the "arc" described.

When a case becomes as complicated as Oscar's, especially when parents have differing viewpoints, and there are complicating psychological components, the pediatrician will often convene a "parent conference" to generate clarity and identify a path forward. That did not happen in this case. My perception was that nothing productive could result from such a meeting. My (total) contact with Oscar's father consisted of one office visit and one phone call in spite of my offering numerous opportunities for him to meet with me. In both situations, he was resistant to my medical recommendations and was overtly rude and critical, making statements like, "you docs are all alike." I ordinarily would have had to prepare for such a conference by soliciting the input of Oscar's psychotherapist but that would have been problematic given the psychotherapist's disinterest in collaborating with me. I was aware also that my senior pediatric partner had a very low opinion of this psychotherapist, and I had seen multiple articles of his in a local parents' newsletter, articles that promoted nutritional solutions for most mental health issues. For these reasons, I did not insist on initiating more regular contact with the psychotherapist and in over 4 years of work with Oscar, he never phoned me or requested that Oscar's mother phone me.

During this period, Oscar's mother phoned me regularly, with statements such as "the psychotherapist thinks Oscar doesn't look well and has recommended a nutritional workup." Because I never spoke with the psychotherapist, I do not know whether Oscar's father was in contact with him and involved in pushing for these workups. My frequent response to Oscar's mother bringing up Oscar's psychotherapist's recommendations was to explain why I did not think a workup or a particular type of treatment was appropriate. His mother was always polite and reasonable and seemed to respect my opinion. Occasionally, I would find out later that a workup (presumably recommended by Oscar's psychotherapist) had been done when I received a set of results and was expected to comment on them. But, she never insisted with me that these recommendations be given priority.

Looking back, these episodes were primarily "irritants." They created extra work and frustration for me. It sometimes felt like I was digging a hole I could never quite get out of, with "sharp objects" occasionally flying up from its depth. But the "do no harm" principle was maintained on all fronts and Oscar did not receive any potentially harmful therapies. There were examples of his mother using what I inferred were strategies for managing the father. Allowing Oscar to be on a gluten-free diet, is an example and seemed to me a clever way to "compromise" on a what I knew could be a disruptive nutritional intervention by father.

As Oscar's medical issues were gradually eclipsed by his psychiatric struggles, my role as "team leader" evolved more into that of a "team member." His therapist made several referrals to child/adolescent psychiatrists. None of them ever initiated contact with me, but I did have a single phone discussion with several of them. I also spoke to the psychologist who assessed Oscar and the head of Special Education at the final public school Oscar attended, following the dangerous bathroom episode. Most importantly, I was ultimately able to strengthen Oscar's mother's case in her confrontation of the school system through a strong letter supporting residential placement; a letter that apparently caused the highest ranking school official to exclaim, "She's on his side!" While it may not have been the school official's intention, to me that comment was a high compliment since it acknowledged that I was fully in support of my patient.

Perhaps my greatest success was in maintaining a cordial and mutually respectful relationship with Oscar's mother who in some sense is the "hero" in this case. Had she not gone to court to obtain full authority over medical decisions, and had she not hired an experienced educational attorney, the course of this case might have been very different. She was uniformly available and appreciative of the time I spent in (not billable) phone discussions regarding problems with Oscar's father or the latest "medical" recommendation from Oscar's psychotherapist. After Oscar's residential placement, she sent e-mails to me and left phone messages at appropriate intervals to report on Oscar's progress, including the diagnosis of his scoliosis and its treatment. Despite the onerous systemic medical, psychiatric, and family issues in this case she never whined; and I never felt she approached me with a selfish or manipulative agenda. Her questions were always about the next step forward for Oscar. Understanding my importance to her, knowing that she and I were joined in a common set of objectives, was probably the biggest source of motivation for me in this very difficult case.

Complexity Summary

1. Biological (including genetic)
   Acute:
   - From early childhood, when treatment was initiated, the patient had multiple acute presentations primarily for allergy related and alleged nutritional problems. Management was in part complicated by disagreements between mother and father about diagnosis, and evidence-based versus untested nutritional interventions. The introduction of an additional, nonmedical provider primarily supported by the patient's father created a significant barrier to implementation of successful, unimpeded treatment.

Chronic:
- The patient had multiple presenting illnesses, both systemic medical and psychiatric. The emotional issues appear to have been significantly fueled by family strife that improved only slowly.

2. Psychiatric/psychological
- The patient was variously described as emotionally compromised, depressed, anxious, and personality disordered. Ultimately the patient presented with psychotic features. His learning impairment appears to have had a psychological basis.

3. Social (including family and other support systems)
- There was a major source of conflict between the future custodial parent (the mother) and the future noncustodial parent (the father). The mother accepted conventional interventions and was supportive of the various physicians treating the patient, whereas the father was help-rejecting and attempted to insert additional mainly unconventional interventions; e.g. laboratory testing, elimination diets, and nutritional supplements none of which were supported by evidence based medicine.

4. Care delivery, including access to care
- The patient/family had access to physicians, laboratory, medications, and other interventions. Care delivery was confounded by father's insistence on unconventional care that frequently was not evidence-based. Care delivery involved a divided system where the mother privately cooperated with the pediatrician and for the most part supported evidence based care

5. Fundamental factors supporting or obstructing the treatment, in particular the quality and continuity of the physician–patient relationship
- In addition to the above, the patient himself for the most part did not resist treatment supported by mother and pediatrician. However he was vociferous about his opposition to many of his father's preferences and requirements. The pediatrician's tireless investment in a long-term treatment relationship with the patient and his mother seems critical to the ultimate success of this patient's care. Her vigor and persistence along with the support of an attorney and educational consultant were instrumental in the school system ultimately accepting the required residential care for Oscar.

Chapter 10
Development of a Major Substance Use Disorder From a Patient's Birth Through His Early Twenties

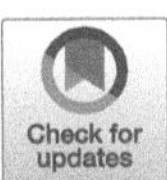

Steven A. Frankel and Jan Maisel

Richard was born at 37+ weeks to an unmarried, teenage mother. His birth weight was 6 pounds, and he had no neonatal problems. He was adopted at birth in an open adoption, with the identity of the biological parents revealed to the adoptive parents from the start.

He was a calm infant, meeting normal growth and developmental milestones. His adoptive parents described him as "loads of fun" as a toddler. He spoke in full sentences by 16 months. He had a good adjustment to daycare and later to school. His parents did, however, experience episodic struggles with Richard around independence and sleeping. When evaluated on at age 6, he was noted to be "slightly impulsive," and his parents said that he was "feisty with limits at times." At age 8, the presenting picture started to change, and he began to report assorted complaints of physical discomfort, all of which made him "anxious."

He was seen at age 10 for a complaint of abdominal pain when away from his parents, thought likely due to homesickness. He also complained of sensing a foreign body in his throat. There were no findings on physical exam. Two months later, he was seen for left testicular pain. Physical exam was again normal. One year later, he was concerned about brief sharp pain in the left rib cage area, occurring "every 2 weeks." His physical exam continued to be benign.

Two years later, at age 13, he experienced an upper respiratory infection (URI) with tracheitis, without fever. Despite absence of fever, this episode led to a prolonged school absence. Four months later, he presented with ongoing "school

S.A. Frankel, MD
Department of Psychiatry, University of California, School of Medicine, San Francisco, CA, USA
e-mail: saf@stevenfrankelmd.com

J. Maisel, MD, PhD (✉)
University of California, Medical Center, San Mateo, CA, USA

Tamalpais Pediatrics, Larkspur, CA, USA
e-mail: janmaisel@gmail.com

© Springer International Publishing AG, part of Springer Nature 2018
S.A. Frankel, J.A. Bourgeois (eds.), *Integrated Care for Complex Patients*,
https://doi.org/10.1007/978-3-319-61214-0_10

problems" including disruptive behaviors, poor academic assignment completion, and excessive absences. He was referred to an experienced child and adolescent psychotherapist. By the end of the school year, his grades had improved.

At age 15, he had a recurrence of more severe testicular pain, and was diagnosed with testicular torsion (an emergent situation). He underwent a successful left testicular torsion repair. Two months later, there was an orthopedic consultation for "one year of left knee pain" and "two weeks of left hip pain." His knee was diagnosed as Osgood-Schlatter disease, a developmental condition that resolves spontaneously. Hip X-ray was normal. MRI revealed no tears, and "small bilateral effusions" not felt to be indicative of a significant problem. A few months later, he was seen for a single unremarkable skin lesion. During this visit, he expressed concern that he was "unhealthy" due to coexisting acne, his diagnosis of Osgood-Schlatter disease, and his prior episodes of hip pain.

Later that year, he was seen by a nurse practitioner for a complaint of anxiety, associated with a rapid heart rate. His school grades were again poor. He was referred for a psychiatric evaluation, resulting in the diagnoses of major depression and generalized anxiety disorder. He was started on escitalopram 20 mg/day. He also presented about this time with very mild pharyngitis, thought by his pediatrician to be a manifestation of globus hystericus (i.e. a psychosomatic condition). His affect was noted to be "glum." Three months later, he was seen for excessive school absences due to "weekly headaches." His parents opted to change high schools with the hope of finding a better fit.

At age 16, he returned to his pediatrician complaining of nausea "off and on for past month." He also reported sporadic vomiting ("six times"), two episodes of diarrhea, and occasional dizziness. He had become dizzy and nauseated and "nearly passed out" at a sporting event. The paramedics were called and reported that his "heart sounded funny" but they did not feel any treatment was needed on site. This "professional opinion" appeared to validate Richard's concerns about his health, and likely led to a significant increase in his level of anxiety.

One month later, Richard's symptoms acutely worsened when on a trip, and he was evaluated at an urgent care facility. On examination, his temperature and EKG were within normal limits. However, his parents did not continue their vacation, feeling that he could not "tolerate" the trip due to his severe anxiety. In his pediatrician's office following this incident his physical exam was benign, but due to an interval 4 pound weight loss laboratory studies were ordered. His laboratory studies included normal results on UA, CBC, and TSH (Thyroid Stimulating Hormone), ESR, CRP (C reactive protein), *H. Pylori* antibody, and celiac testing, all of which were negative. He also was referred for psychometric testing, the results of which revealed very good cognitive skills. He did, however, show some difficulty in reading comprehension, focus, and other executive functions, and findings consistent with depression and low self-esteem.

Some months later, he awoke one morning with right neck pain. X-ray in an emergency department revealed "straightening of normal cervical lordosis consistent with muscle spasm." He was given a cervical collar, diazepam, and ibuprofen. Within 1 month, he returned to clinic stating that his neck symptoms recurred upon return to school, and he was given additional diazepam. He was seen a month later for persistent neck pain. Decreased range of motion (ROM) had persisted. An orthopedic consultant felt that a new X-ray showed "pathological straightening of normal spinal curve." The orthopedic consultant had prescribed the patient diazepam 5 mg BID and acetaminophen/hydrocodone every 6–8 h. The patient was subsequently able to attend school on these medications. He had a second orthopedic appointment at which these medications were continued. It is noteworthy that his parents viewed this episode as the one that started his later addictions. At this point, he began psychotherapy with a psychologist specializing in cognitive behavioral therapy. His psychiatrist prescribed buspirone for anxiety but the patient complained that he had a "bad reaction" to the medication, paradoxically in the form of increased anxiety resulting in several missed days of school.

A subsequent neck CT (Computerized Axial Tomography) scan was unremarkable and physical therapy was recommended. He requested more diazepam and was given a small supply. Soon thereafter, he began a taper of acetaminophen/hydrocodone and diazepam. Six weeks later, his neck pain had resolved. He was seen 1 month later for complaint of difficulty falling asleep at night and frequent awakening, despite newly prescribed 30 mg mirtazapine each night. He claimed the sleeping problem was causing intermittent school absence. The patient felt that his insomnia was due to recent onset of left upper back/shoulder pain that was poorly responsive to ibuprofen. He also saw a chiropractor, but stated that treatment provided only very transient relief ("15 minutes"). Physical exam revealed mild tenderness along medial border left scapula.

In a subsequent phone conversation with the patient's mother his issues included anxiety ("he never feels physically good") and refusal to work with his CBT therapist, the patient having stated: "I want a pill to make the pain go away." He was unable to keep up with academic demands, necessitating a transfer to an alternative high school for students unable to manage the requirements of a mainstream high school program.

When seen in clinic that month, he presented with scapular pain that he claimed had been persistent since his last visit. The pain was described as a "spasm" and a "pulling sensation" between his shoulder blade and mid-back. He had been prescribed (but had not taken) ibuprofen as he felt it did not help his pain and was disruptive of sleep. He had also recently stopped taking prescribed sleep medication as he felt he was getting headaches from it. He also continued to complain of anxiety, and had not yet taken the methylphenidate recently prescribed by the psychiatrist to address his attentional problems.

During this time, Richard had an orthopedic appointment with normal x-rays of his chest and spine. The orthopedic surgeon did not find anything that could explain the Richard's pain and speculated that the pain was due to muscle spasm. His mother reported that her son was "withdrawing, spending all his time downstairs in a dark room watching TV" and falling behind in school. Tension at home was at a peak, leading the patient, in frustration, to throw a bottle of pills at his mother crying, "no one knows how to help me."

Richard's mother felt that the family was now "in crisis." Richard was refusing to continue to see the chiropractor who had been treating him or to try massage "because it will hurt too much." He further insisted that he could not do "any" exercise. He stated, "I want to go to school but I'm in too much pain to go to school until someone finds out what's wrong with my back." He was not regularly attending school, with the school system considering mandated withdrawal from school and initiation of home schooling. The parents believed he was "in pain," but they were out of ideas and running out of money. As a measure of the stress the situation was causing, at this point, the patient's father sought psychiatric care because of his own suicidal thoughts.

The following is a statement from his pediatrician's notes at this time: "I feel the focus now needs to be on managing the patient's symptoms and doubt any additional tests are indicated." The orthopedist treating him has recommended an acupuncture trial that he said might work for muscle pain. He also recommended a consult with a university-based pediatric pain service." His pediatrician strongly recommended to parents that they impose consequences of no car or TV access if Richard did not attend school. The patient's mother requested that a muscle relaxant be prescribed for Richard, and a 2-week supply of cyclobenzaprine was ordered.

Two months later, the pain was "much better," now "minimal" in the back and neck area. However, Richard reported that panic attacks were occurring frequently. The psychiatrist prescribed small amounts of clonazepam for these. The parents also decided to cancel his pain clinic appointment because they were convinced that anxiety was the "cause of his discomfort."

At this point, at age 17, Richard left the public school setting for home schooling and agreed to resume psychotherapy. He was also hired as a part-time assistant in a local real estate office. His parents engaged a tutor plus an educational counselor. The overriding focus for the parents was "preserving the family unit since it was in such disarray." Consistently, the parents reported that they had resolved to stop "reacting" and had decided to allow Richard to "find his own path." Although this shift of posture seemed quite logical, unfortunately it was associated with a sharp exacerbation in Richard's difficulties, with frank addiction becoming manifest from this point. It is worth noting that this kind of sequence is familiar in the treatment of addicted youth.

Later that year, Richard's mother called his pediatrician to report the discovery that he had become addicted to oxycodone and clonazepam. The parents enrolled him in an inpatient rehabilitation program. He appeared to do well in the program initially by saying "the right things in order to get out quickly." However, his manipulations failed and he remained for 70 days. The parents additionally participated in a week-long educational program on addiction for themselves, which they felt was extremely helpful for understanding Richard's condition.

Psychological testing while in rehabilitation pointed to obsessive–compulsive disorder (OCD) and panic disorder. According to the report, much of Richard's anxiety was expressed in "body symptoms," based on his worries about his health. Both received therapeutic attention. He was tried (without effect) on sertraline

100 mg/day. Upon returning home, he was referred to Narcotics Anonymous and started working with an addiction specialist. During this time, drug testing was temporarily clean, and he began attending classes at a private school. Four months later, Richard reported recurrent neck pain, and he again was prescribed cyclobenzaprine and diazepam. He soon relapsed to abusing oxycodone and was referred for inpatient substance abuse rehabilitation, after which he was lost to followup for a period of time.

Two years later, his parents reported that he had been in a new rehabilitation program (primarily for oxycodone abuse) for a year. Initially, he was assigned to an inpatient unit, then moved to a "less restrictive" environment until he was living on his own in an apartment near his parents' home. He was working in a shop and had begun taking classes at a community college. The unfortunate time delays between primary care visits were noted. These delays are common in primary care where lapses in treatment and provider changes may occur for idiosyncratic reasons such as insurance denials.

Four months later, in a phone conversation with the patient's mother, the pediatrician learned that Richard had attempted to relocate to another state to "start his life over with his birth family" and began to use drugs again while there. He sustained two concussions under mysterious circumstances during this period. He left the hospital against medical advice after the first concussion, refusing to see a neurologist. His mother flew to meet him and drive him back to California. After the second concussion, he agreed to see a local neurologist. On examination she found dysmetria, intention tremor, neck and back spasm, and postconcussion syndrome. A brain MRI (magnetic resonance imaging) was ordered, and he was sent to physical therapy. However, his pediatrician felt that the neurologist missed the somatization/anxiety-related aspects of his symptoms.

Six months later, in another telephone call with his mother, it was learned that Richard had again relapsed into oxycodone abuse. He voluntarily went to detoxification and rehabilitation for 2 weeks and then was discharged on buprenorphine for maintainance of opiate withdrawal. At this point his mother began a 18-month academic program in drug addiction counseling. Over time, she arrived at the conviction that Richard had suffered from overwhelming anxiety since age 3, and that his "adoption was the biggest wound." Sadly, at the present time Richard's prognosis remains uncertain. The saga continues with Richard, and his family battling the tenacious, unforgiving menace of addiction.

Pediatrician's Reflections

Additional thoughts on Richard from the perspective of his PCP:

During Richard's early years, each of his physical symptoms was straightforwardly dealt with in office visits with me. At these visits, I provided ample reassurance for both Richard and his parents. However, because I was made aware of developments only once a year, neither Richard's parents nor I could fully grasp the "bigger picture" of his escalating anxiety and unrelenting obsessional symptoms. It is likely that his parents were not capable of generating this perspective as Richard was their first/only child and their responses were nurturing and problem solving, not analytical. Their sensitivity about his adoption might have been another factor in his parents' inability to step back and gain perspective about his developing difficulties.

The onset of both academic and behavioral problems was a red flag to me. I responded by referring Richard to one of the most skilled psychotherapists I knew. There was initial improvement, but it halted and his mood and physical symptoms worsened significantly during the following 18 months. It was also extremely difficult for me to tease out what was medically significant for explaining school absences and underachievement. Thus began a flurry of orthopedic referrals, both pediatric and adult. It was the initial opiate prescription by the adult orthopedist that his parents feel set Richard on the road toward addiction.

I do not have a clear sense of how early the issue of Richard's adoption was experienced as a wound by him. It certainly was an ever-present background issue. Statements made during his checkups confirmed telephone contact with his birth family occurring at least yearly. I believe that there were also visits with several birth family members during this period.

After the diagnosis of substance abuse was finally made my involvement with this case became peripheral. The parents stepped in beautifully and worked with addiction specialists at multiple rehabilitation programs over the ensuing 4 years. During this period, they learned to set appropriate limits on Richard's behaviors thereby forestalling relapses. I have a great deal of respect for the love, dedication, and persistence in their fierce dedication to their son.

Complexity Summary

1. Biological (including genetic)
   Acute:
   - The treatment report covers period from adoption and infancy to age 20. It traces development of anxiety and overreaction by Richard to minor physical ailments through the evolution of addiction to opioids.
   Chronic:
   - Over time, this patient's course was marked by pain, depression, OCD, anxiety, and ultimately addiction.
2. Psychiatric/psychological
   - Psychiatric comorbidity was at least partially centered around unresolved adoption (and parenting) issues. While this is an inference, support comes from Richard's decision to temporarily move to live with his biological parents at age 20.
   - This formulation, however, is complicated and his adoption based anxiety could have been superseded by the patient's addiction to benzodiazepines and

opioids. In these types of circumstances, it is often impossible to discern basic psychopathology. When addiction is involved it often disrupts and overshadows ordinary psychological life.

3. Social (including family and other support systems)
   - Richard's adoptive family was loving and attentive. His abuse of substances suggests a need to self-medicate to contain his anxiety and obsessionality, as well as mitigate his personal and social confusion. This pattern is often encountered with adopted children and may reflect issues associated with a shaky sense of identity (do I truly belong in my family? who am I really?).

4. Care delivery, including access to care
   - The family had full access to and used a full spectrum of high-quality medical and psychiatric care including specialists in addiction. When new issues cropped up, new personnel and approaches were tried including CBT (cognitive behavioral therapy), coaching, and teaching home-based measures.

5. Fundamental factors supporting or obstructing the treatment, in particular quality and continuity of the physician–patient relationship
   - One possibility for explaining Richard's vulnerability to addiction is that Richard's parents may have been overly solicitous with him, focusing on his claimed physical problems from childhood. Studies suggest that parents of adopted children often attempt to "make up for the adoption" by being overly attentive to their adopted children, as if the fundamental felt "defect" of the adoption can be repaired in that way. Paradoxically this behavior may communicate to the child that the parents believe he or she is in fact defective, "special" but in a negative way. Logically, the harder these parents try to compensate for the feared damage created by the adoption, the more likely they are to fuel the problem by confirming the child's uncertainty about his or her legitimacy. Treatment of these cases requires psychological sophistication and skills beyond that of the typical primary care physician.
   - Citation — Frankel, S. (1991), Pathogenic Factors in the Experience of Early and Late Adopted children. The Psychoanalytic Study of the Child, 46:91–108.

Chapter 11
Two Adolescent Brothers with Postviral Encephalitis Neurological Syndrome and Associated Psychological Overlay involving Parental Enmeshment

J. Richard Mendius

The complexities of this case center on two brothers, Philip and Mark, and their analogous symptoms. Both brothers appeared to have parallel cognitive and emotional disorders without clear etiologies ever established. Viral and other infectious illnesses were put forward as putative causes but without any clear evidence that these were actually the etiological agents. Both boys were initially seen for assessment of a probable postinfectious encephalopathy or an autoimmune reaction associated with a streptococcal pharyngitis. Although there was no family history of cognitive or psychiatric illness, some genetic underpinning had to be entertained until proven otherwise. Philip, age 15, presented first. His brother Mark, age 13, was initially seen 7 months later. Complicating this picture is the suspicion of interpersonal complicity among the boys and their parents, encouraging the mirroring of symptoms.

Also involved in obscuring the clarity of the findings and their etiology is the erratic nature of the consultation process with several primary care physicians and medical specialists, including myself providing consultation to the parents. For the most part, I was involved as a consultant, but at times I needed to make medical decisions independently acknowledging that these were being rendered outside of my role as consultant. My official role, however, was that of a consulting neurologist and my involvement in the case was, of necessity, intermittent.

This case involves two adolescent brothers who initially suffered from what was assumed to be postviral encephalitis accompanied by balance, concentration, memory, and fine motor impairments. Over time, systemic medical indicators were only mildly supportive. Over time, the similarity between the symptoms experienced by both boys underscored the probability of an ongoing psychiatric etiology, associated with parental encouragement and enmeshment.

J. Richard Mendius (✉)
Sutter Pacific Medical Center, Santa Rosa, CA, USA
e-mail: jrichardmendius@aol.com

© Springer International Publishing AG, part of Springer Nature 2018
S.A. Frankel, J.A. Bourgeois (eds.), *Integrated Care for Complex Patients*,
https://doi.org/10.1007/978-3-319-61214-0_11

I was consulted late in the development of the case after multiple evaluations by local physicians and neurology specialists at major medical academic centers. I was consulted as a physician who might "think out of the box."

Patient #1, Philip

Philip was an ambidextrous Caucasian male in excellent health until age 15 when he developed a flu-like illness with continued malaise for 3 months. At that time, he reported cognitive compromise, which he described as an "inner blackness." This event was accompanied by ataxia, stuttering, paraphasic errors, dysmnesia (distortion of memory), and migraine headaches, which were intractable. He also complained of right thigh pain. The patient's parents refused neuropsychological consultation at this time.

Laboratory data included a 24-hour EEG monitor, which showed no abnormalities. He had a PET scan showing 5% reduction in biparietal metabolism. An MRI of the brain showed left periventricular white matter changes, particularly in the left centrum semiovale, both frontal and parietal. His past medical history was positive for a GI hemorrhage without apparent sequelae. Family history included an inclusion body myositis for the maternal grandfather.

When first seen, Philip was on no prescription medications. His general examination was unremarkable. His neurological exam was positive only for slowed cognition and depressed affect. My initial speculation was that he likely had CNS demyelination in the left centrum semiovale, possible residual scarring from viral encephalitis, and a possible ongoing inflammatory condition such as pediatric autoimmune neuropsychiatric disorder (PANDAS), associated with a streptococcus infection. There were a combination of ambigous findings that also suggested past traumatic brain injury including flattening of the prefrontal pole with decreased metabolic activity in the cerebellum, parietal, and occipital areas. However, there was no reported history of head trauma (for either of the brothers). A later MRI of the brain showed equivocal residual frontal lobe scarring.

Philip was relatively passive about his condition. He was quite aware of his unusual combination of cognitive and depressive symptoms, but felt helpless about influencing them. His lack of emotionality was striking. His lack of initiative extended to most aspects of his life, including schoolwork, with his illness progressively interfering with his school attendance.

Philip was at first treated without success with a dihydroergotamine (DHE) protocol for medically refractory migraine and cluster headache. He was evaluated at an academic medical center and diagnosed as having the residua of viral encephalitis. He gradually improved from with remaining autobiographical amnesia, anosmia, and cognitive dysfunction. Unfortunately, he began to decline again, developing such a severe (apparant) memory loss that he could only retain events for a few hours. According to reports from the parents, this development was also accompanied by difficulty recognizing words, acalculia, lack of number recognition, and "loss of recognition of the world around him." A neuropsychological assessment at that time was essentially unremarkable. This situation persisted through 2007 when he was extensively reevaluated at a world-class referral center distant from his home. Surprisingly, he received the relatively benign diagnoses of "severe sleep disturbance with delayed sleep phase syndrome (DSPS), and postural orthostatic tachycardia syndrome (POTS)."

He returned to me 2 years after my first evaluation for another consultation, and drawing on accumulating evidence I began to entertain "limbic encephalitis residua" as his main diagnosis and started him on valganciclovir (an antiviral drug effective with cytomegalovirus). Thereafter, he appeared to improve. Referring to possible visuospatial (parietal lobe) improvement, his mother commented that complex card games were easier for him to do than other cognitive chores. When asked, Philip noted that strategy card games were similar to strategies he had learned from computer games.

Three months later he was switched from valganciclovir to famciclovir, antiviral medications that target different viruses. He underwent a quantitative electroencephalography, which showed abnormal spectral analysis. EEG assisted rehabilitation and neural biofeedback were attempted at this point. However, the patient reported that the most helpful remediation came from working with his teachers, a course of neural optometric treatment, and reading rehabilitation[1,2,3].

He had a mild balance disturbance, mild hand apraxia, and marked difficulty playing guitar, a musical instrument he had previously mastered. Of note, in contrast with his previous abilities, he could not picture a musical piece or video game sequence although he could execute the required muscle movements.

Later that year, it was noted that the patient was able to use a computer mouse with either hand and was playing a keyboard for bimanual music effects. Neurofeedback, biofeedback, cognitive rehabilitation, and sleep hygiene counseling were continued. The patient was tried with multiple medications including gabapentin and duloxetine for pain and hyperbaric oxygen to facilitate resolution of inferred encephalitis.

---

[1] Quantitative electroencephalography (qEEG) is a procedure that processes the recorded EEG activity from a multielectrode recording using a computer. The qEEG is an extension of the analysis of the visual EEG interpretation which may assist and even augment our understanding of the EEG and brain function.

[2] Power spectral analysis is a well-established method for the analysis of EEG signals. Spectral parameters can be used to quantify pharmacological effects.

[3] Neuro-optometric rehabilitation is a therapy that utilizes optometric vision therapy, prisms, lenses, filters, and occlusion to help stimulate parts of the brain, which are not functioning to their highest potential due to interruptions caused by brain injury. Brain injury may result from concussion, stroke, birth trauma (ADD/ADHD), chemical trauma (chemotherapy), physical trauma, and in-utero trauma (cerebral palsy, fetal alchol syndrome.)

However, within months, he again regressed with the loss of previous memory and mathematical dysfunction. I lost track of him for the next year and half. When he returned for an appointment, he was continuing to struggle with his schoolwork and complained of constant headaches and right eye pain, sleep dysregulation, and memory problems. He felt as though his brain was "ten steps ahead of his hands." He would play video games but found it hard to move the cursor and joysticks. He was more effective with his right hand than his left, and his right thumb was more facile than his left. He also reported that processing and remembering information were exceedingly difficult for him.

At points during this period of treatment, Philip had also been receiving alternative treatments at a local neuropsychiatry center and treatments for neurorehabilitation at a major medical center both arranged by his parents and not directly reported to me. His parents also arranged for hyperbaric oxygen treatments (HBOT). There is tentative evidence for the efficacy of HBOT in neurorehabilitation for traumatic brain injury [1]. In 2011, some improvement was noted in chronological association with the hyperbaric oxygen treatment. Nonetheless, he reported being constantly exhausted, needing to take frequent breaks from schoolwork.

At this point, my involvement in Philip's care ceased. As mentioned, my role in this case was that of consultant and I was not retained in the treatment in spite of frequent follow-up reminders sent by my office. Equally, except for making suggestions, I was not successful at introducing appropriate specialists into the treatment, including mental health professionals. The absence of follow-up to Philip's story is likely reflective of the fragmentation of care that often characterizes the US care delivery system. Transfers of providers occur frequently, often disrupting continuity of care. The causes are manifold but often insurance provisions are shifted, so that the providers do not remain available or the fee structure is changed discouraging patients from continuing the care. It is also important that this family was simultaneously consulting with more than one primary care provider (PCP) and several specialists, and that these practitioners were not collaborating with one another, thereby undermining the possibility of realizing a consistent treatment.

Patient #2, Mark

At presentation, 6 months after Philip sought my help, Philip's brother Mark was referred to me for treatment. At that time, Mark was a 13-year-old right-handed Caucasian male. He had been in excellent health until age 13, when he developed a streptococcus pharyngitis. He was treated with antibiotics and within 3 months developed an ASO titer of 690 units. He later developed polyarthralgias, lymphadenopathy, and was treated with penicillin and nonsteroidal anti-inflammatory agents. He underwent adenotonsillectomy with some benefit. Two years later, he had a two-week upper respiratory infection and woke with a right eye central scotoma associated with ocular pain. The areas of visual deficit were described by him initially as "black" but within 8 hours as "smoky." He was seen by ophthalmology without a diagnosis being established. However, he had an elevated Epstein-Barr virus titer and was started on valganciclovir. He continued to have visual aberrations and painful lymphadenopathy.

Three months later, Mark developed neurological symptoms analogous to those of his brother, including stumbling, word-finding problems, insomnia, cognitive decline, short-term memory dysfunction, episodes of loss of awareness, and inability to read due to the loss of ability to maintain focus on the words. Once again, the family did not follow through with recommended neuropsychological testing. He was noted to have an elevated HHV-6 titer. He developed "tingling" in both upper and both lower extremities, vertigo with lightheadedness, stomach pain, and nausea. He was noted to have an elevated opening pressure on the lumbar puncture and was placed on acetazolamide. This treatment did not change his symptoms.

When he was seen during the next year, he was complaining of headaches of an "8–9.5 out of 10" intensity, generalized painful lymphadenopathy, intermittent eye pain, worsening memory and cognition, and progressive difficulty sleeping. He found it hard to do homework because of apparent cognitive slowing, difficulty with concentration, and fatigue. He had no incontinence, paralysis, numbness, or gait ataxia. At this point, he was carrying the diagnoses of mild cognitive impairment, attention-deficit disorder without hyperactivity, frontal lobe executive function deficit, and postural orthostatic tachycardia syndrome. He also complained of intermittent periods of depression.

His physical exam showed some tender small nodes in his neck but otherwise was unremarkable. His neurological exam was positive for slowed speech and depressed affect but no other gross neurobehavioral dysfunction. His cranial nerve, motor, sensory, cerebellar, gait, and deep tendon reflexes were unremarkable. Formal neuropsychological testing, laboratory data from cerebrospinal fluid, and a structural/functional SPECT scan were ordered. The testing never occurred, however, as the parents never followed through. The SPECT scan showed medial thalamic and basal ganglia activity increase consistent with anxiety and depression. It also showed anterior cingulate and lateral prefrontal increase with concentration, and difficulties shifting attention with a rigidity of thought processes. It was noted that the left and right temporal lobes did not activate with concentration, which was felt to be consistent with an auditory processing problem and learning disability. There was decreased function in the inferior frontal lobes consistent with those attributed to attention-deficit disorder and in the cerebellum correlated with difficulties with complex motor acts and with frontal lobe memory consolidation.

He was referred by his parents to a physician practicing complementary medicine and was treated with tyrosine allegedly for supplementation of dopamine and phenylalanine as well as supplementation of norepinephrine, phosphatidylserine, fish oil, and S-adenosyl methionine (SAMe). I prescribed duloxetine for his depressive symptoms. He began cognitive retraining. In consultation with another physician, his parents started him on treatment with hyperbaric oxygen, presumably for his cognitive dysfunction. Neuropsychological testing also showed slowed processing speed and frontal lobe dysfunction. He was evaluated for a sleep phase disorder and tried unsuccessfully on eszopiclone.

He had some return of his cognitive function within a few months and was able to finish his semester at school. When seen 3 months later, he was continuing to have some problems with headaches, fatigue, sleep, and "clear thinking." An EEG showed paroxysmal discharges in the temporal lobe, and the patient was started on lamotrigine. A repeat SPECT scan showed improvement. On a combination of lamotrigine, duloxetine and adjunctive treatments, the patient was able to improve his intellectual function and start attending school at a community college.

Commentary by Author

Mark's case suffered the same fate as that of his brother, Philip. After the initial round of consultations, he disappeared from my practice. The reason for his leaving, as with Philip, is unknown to me. Possibilities in both cases included spontaneous remission of the boys' symptoms, medical insurance complications, changes influencing choice and availability of primary care physician and/or consultant, or dissatisfaction with my care. The reason remains obscure. What does seem likely as a potential source of parental dissatisfaction, however, is that in addition to systemic medical causes there was a major psychiatric component to the boys' presenting illnesses. This contribution was never formally identified or addressed. The parents assiduously resisted entertaining the possibility of a psychiatric explanation for a presentation that in both cases was originally considered to be medical in character, that is, as reflecting a postviral syndrome. Presumably, the parents conspired in creating and maintaining what was essentially a folie a duex involving the brothers, an interpersonal process in which the people involved are so closely aligned with each other that they share aspects of their personalities, each acting and ostensibly feeling like the other. In this case, there seems to have been parental support for such a process.

My own observation, not as well documented as I would like, is that there was indeed "complicity" between the brothers as they joined their beliefs about their illnesses. Supporting this process, the parents exerted great pressure to identify a "cause… any cause" for the boys' medical and psychiatric presentations. Central to the fragmentation in this case was also the inability of the family and primary care physicians to join in a sufficiently consistent union.

Of particular relevance is the level of frustration I experienced in attempting to do my part in the treatment of this case. It is notable that support services including speech therapy, cognitive therapy, and psychological services were instrumental in keeping this case moving forward. For me, the case raises the vexing problem of work with a family that has extensive resources but for whom cure was elusive. Unable to find the solutions they desired locally and within their arbitrary time frame, they invoked the illusion that they could purchase the miraculous cure they were intent on receiving and repeatedly transferred care in order to obtain the cure they sought.

Complexity Summary

1. Biological
   Acute:
   - Presumably both boys initially suffered from a postviral encephalitis accompanied by balance, concentration, memory, and fine motor impairments. Over time, systemic medical indicators were mildly supportive but equivocal. The similarity between the symptoms experienced by both boys underscores the probability of an ongoing psychiatric etiology. No significant environmental stressors were identified.

   Chronic:
   - One possible explanation for the observed course is conversion from an acute neurological condition to a chronic one, although the time frame seems short for such a process. Ongoing psychological mechanisms involving family complicity seem more likely.
2. Psychiatric/psychological
   - There was never a clear diagnosis of specific psychiatric illness in these cases. Both of these cases involved adolescents. According to the author of this case narrative, of central importance was "family pathology associated with hyper-involved parents, who served as the ringmasters for what appears to be a family generated medical drama." "The parents' anxiety/fear/suffering about losing their "perfect children" are seen by him as instrumental for understanding these cases. He goes on to say that, "An earlier psychiatric intervention involving a coordinating psychiatrist, engaged at the behest of the boys' pediatrician, might have saved this case. Illustrated is the peril of not having a health provider in a central, coordinating role that could block such a development."
3. Social (including family and other support systems)
   - Unlike more typical cases where the support system is weak or missing, in this case it was powerful and in ways impenetrable. The parents in this case were presumably instrumental in orchestrating and maintaining pathology-based developments and unresponsive to interventions directed at curbing them
4. Care delivery, including access to care
   - Apparently intact. No clear restrictions in access to care. In fact, it may have been the families' extensive financial resources that were problematic for treatment. With extensive financial means to support care, they were able to take full advantage of all conventional and alternative medical resources. The

latter were often substituted for conventional treatments, at times handicapping the progress of the case.

5. Fundamental factors supporting or obstructing the treatment, in particular the quality and continuity of the physician–patient relationship
   - Exclusion of a central PCP, from consistent involvement in this case and the parents' insistence on managing the case according to their wishes, defeated the possibility of the development of a viable physician/patient–family bond.
   - This is a scenario that is encountered frequently in primary care, people signing up for only the care they understand and desire, consulting with friends and unqualified health care providers about what clinical steps should be taken. The author of this narrative is very experienced and skilled and, if supported, undoubtly could have guided this case to a successful conclusion.

Reference

1. Kranke P, Bennett MH, Martyn-St James M, Schnabel A, Debus SE, Weibel S. Hyperbaric Oxygen Therapy for Treating Chronic Wounds. Cochrane Library; 2015.

Chapter 12
An Adolescent Boy with Allergic Sensitivity and Anaphylaxis as an Infant, Crippling Parental Overprotection, and Unconfirmed Epilepsy

J. Richard Mendius and Steven A. Frankel

Barton initially presented to my neurology clinic for evaluation at age 14. He had a number of complicated neurological and psychiatric symptoms that required multi-specialty management, neuroimaging, and video/EEG telemetry. He was the second child born of parents in their late 30's. Prior to his concurrent combined psychiatric–psychotherapy treatment, he had been in treatment with multiple mental health professionals including psychiatrists and nonmedical psychotherapists.

The patient's medical symptoms began at birth when he was delivered by C-section for fetal bradycardia. Beginning about the age of 4, he was discovered to "respond poorly to noxious environmental stimuli," which resulted in his parents protectively isolating him from contact with other children. His physical development was relatively normal but his speech function was delayed until age 3 when it thereafter quickly progressed to normal. He had a concussion at age 4, which was uncomplicated and was not worked up with neuroimaging or EEG and required no further treatment.

From this point, Barton's parents, frightened for his health and safety, began to monitor his every move. His father, in particular, knew every detail about his habits as if he alone could assure that his already "damaged" child would live a life without any further harm, physically or emotional.

When Barton began his education at age 6, he was reported to have a great deal of difficulty with school performance in large part based on his high level of anxiety, restlessness. Simultaneously, he avoided most social contacts. Both Barton and his

J. Richard Mendius (✉)
Sutter Pacific Medical Center, Santa Rosa, CA, USA
e-mail: jrichardmendius@aol.com

S.A. Frankel, MD (✉)
Department of Psychiatry, University of California, School of Medicine, San Francisco, CA, USA
e-mail: saf@stevenfrankelmd.com

S.A. Frankel, J.A. Bourgeois (eds.), *Integrated Care for Complex Patients*,
https://doi.org/10.1007/978-3-319-61214-0_12

parents supported Barton's self-concept as medically and psychologically damaged by alleging that he could not tolerate the lack of sensitivity of the behavior of his peers.

Beginning about age 8, Barton developed multiple motor tics and some obsessional behaviors including touching rituals and word repetitions. Included were eye blinking, head shrugging, facial grimacing (both unilateral and bilateral), grunting with vocalizations such as "grr," hiccups, clicks, and growls. These behaviors decreased when Barton became engrossed in a task. They were not controlled with benzodiazepines, alpha-2 adrenergic agents (e.g., clonidine), psychostimulants, or serotonin reuptake inhibitors. Barton's parents were generally resistant to conventional medications including psychotropics and simultaneously pursued "alternative" treatments including vitamin Bl, folic acid, iron, fish oil, kava, and calcium. All of these treatments except probiotics reportedly failed to help contain Barton's "hyperactivity" and anxiety.

Barton's parents, although presumably seeking effective treatment, were clearly in accord with Barton's view of himself as "damaged" and reinforced his conviction that he was "medically at risk." As an observer it was difficult to tell whether and when the reported behaviors had a true medical basis. Barton's claim that he could not manage in school and socially was accepted unconditionally by his parents. Each new symptom, each claimed exacerbation, gleaned support. Hence, while ostensibly wanting the best for him, Barton's parents were progressively handicapping him.

Originally, Barton was the best resource for distinguishing between his "anxiety symptoms" and those that had a medical explanation. However, over time, through his adolescence, Barton also lost perspective, and the originally perceptive Barton progressively lost hope and stopped trying to "understand" ("after all what good will it do, my parents will make more rules for me"). Of note is that during this period Barton had been in the care of several psychiatrists for anxiety, depression, suicidality, and tic disorder.

When Barton first presented, he reported a several month history of "flashing light" sensations over his occiput and temples. These were accompanied by combined jerking–convulsing–screaming behavior. He also developed episodes of "severe anxiety" preventing him from socializing or attending school. These episodes were in part characterized by pervasive pessimism and anxiety, building at times to panic. This progression of symptoms started after an episode of viral encephalitis at age 13 for which he was hospitalized. Of note, he refused to attend school for 4 months following this hospitalization. He reported to his parents and to me (R.M.) that he felt as though "all the electrical energy" in his brain was "concentrated" in those anxious periods. He had photophobia but no other migrainous symptoms and he had a negative ASO titer.

Subsequent to this episode, Barton had an extensive metabolic workup, with negative testing for Lyme disease and CMV serology studies for Epstein-Barr, which were consistent with a past exposure without a current infection. His initial neurological exam was unremarkable except for equivocal bilateral hyporeflexia and multiple vocalizations throughout the exam, most of which were suppressible. He was scheduled for MRI of the brain and an EEG. The MRI was unremarkable.

However, later that year, before he was able to have his EEG, Barton had the first of his "epileptic" events. The patient was riding his bicycle and apparently collapsed with bilateral upper and lower extremity shaking movements consistent with a generalized tonic–clonic seizure lasting approximately 90 seconds in duration. Later, he recalled a lapse of memory and some confusion including an inability to recall his name. He had ingested nothing more than one Ibuprofen capsule approximately an hour before the event. There were no motor coordination problems.

He was brought to an emergency department. A CT scan of his brain was negative, and an EEG showed some right temporal slowing. It was suggested in the ER that he start on levetiracetam, but discussion with the family about potential side effects caused them to refuse to comply, which then resulted in a trial of divalproex sodium that was stopped when it caused ataxia,. Ultimately, he responded to lamotrigine for both mood stabilization and seizure control. Lamotrigine was slowly increased to 200 mg/day.

Despite anticonvulsant treatment, the patient continued to have of the claimed "seizures" that gradually increased in frequency. At age 15, he was having weekly episodes, which persisted despite a trial of lacosimide. The seizures were described as involving an aura of dizziness and vertigo accompanied by sensation of separation from his surroundings. This state was followed by a loss of consciousness with closed eyes, hypersalivation, and symmetrical bilateral upper extremity tremor progressing to lower extremity. There were multiple "triggers" he believed were responsible for the seizures including physical activity such as running, emotional upset, pain, and startling noises. Of interest, his parents had originally described Barton as "hypersensitive," unable to tolerate "buzzing" noises.

Because of the long-standing history of school failure, neuropsychological testing was initiated. Quoting from the neuropsychology testing report, "… paradoxically his assessment revealed numerous strengths. He tested as highly intelligent with a potential for bringing to bear sophisticated psychological coping resources. He showed a high need for achievement. He could quickly understand and integrate different complex abstract verbal and visual-spatial concepts."

His scores on measures of verbal reasoning, fluid visuospatial reasoning, and auditory working memory were in the high average to superior range. One of his scores, that measured fluid spatial reasoning, was at the 89th percentile rank for his age. He was also above average in performance on measures of reading and in remembering verbal material presented within a meaningful context such as a story.

In contrast to these strengths, Barton's assessment demonstrated noteworthy difficulties in select areas of attention and executive functioning. His attention span was inconsistent. This variability was attributed to fluctuations in affect and in coping operations as well as difficulties in maintaining focus. With respect to his executive functions, he was found to be capable of initiating and coming up with strategies for problem-solving. Mathematics was a personal strength. However, he was "often slower than expected while preforming, shifting mental sets during problem solving tasks."

Barton's behavior during assessment sessions as well as his results on measures of mood, behavior, and personality, revealed numerous strengths including, ironically, a positive sense of humor. "He can be very perceptive, talkative, and friendly when he interacts with others, especially adults. However, his results across all methods of assessment revealed frequent episodes of intense anxious-depressed affect". It was concluded that a core problem for Barton was a "very poor self-concept." In Barton's words, "I am a misfit and that's the way it is." According to the assessing psychologist, "his deficient, fragmented self-concept will make it hard for him to arrive at personal strategies to progress in life, as well as to initiate and maintain close friendships. He is not presently at risk for self-harm but that risk level could quickly increase if current sources of social and emotional support were suddenly removed from him."

Barton required an individual education plan (IEP) for his schooling in part because he was only intermittently attending class. Amphetamine/dextroamphetamine 5 mg was started in an attempt to improve his school performance. On his first day taking it, Barton had an event involving opisthotonic-like posturing i.e. generalized extension of the trunk and lower limbs with increased muscular tone. If nothing else, this development was extremely dramatic.

In spite of a rapid return to normal and in response to his parents' insistence, Barton's medications to aid with focusing were sequentially and impulsively changed. Trials included buproprion, lisdexamphetaime, dexmethylphenidate, and escitalopram, all without success. Side effects including increased anxiety were repeatedly cited as the reason for his treatment failures.

When seen at age 15, Barton reported eight events (all of which he called "seizures") over the previous 3 months. One occurred when playing soccer and another when swimming. He was disturbed by the number of "seizure" events, his inability to enjoy activities because of the sudden onset of these events, and his refractoriness to treatment with either stimulants or anticonvulsants. Note, however, it was unclear to multiple examiners whether the patient actually had electrical epilepsy as opposed to psychogenic nonelectric epilepsy-like events (PNES). However, his parents never failed to view the events as classical epilepsy, and they acted accordingly.

Barton was referred for a video EEG telemetry recording to capture clinical and behavioral events. The initial EEG showed a posterior dominant rhythm of 7–8 Hz, with frequent high-amplitude but irregular generalized spike and slow wave discharges. A single seizure was captured, but the patient was off camera in the rest room at the time of the reported event. Prior to the onset of the "seizure" the EEG was characterized by a prolonged run of monomorphic moderate to high amplitude theta and delta activity, followed by high-amplitude generalized frontally predominant irregular sharp activity. The patient indicated multiple events of dizziness, which were not definitively associated with the interictal discharges described above. He also described visual abberations but these were not associated with any change in the background EEG rhythm. It was felt – albeit not established – that the patient did indeed have generalized convulsive seizures, and that he had multiple other events, which were nonictal.

The patient was never able to get below the described seizure frequency of one per week when on lamotrigine. He was then transitioned to valproate but without significant benefit and with side effects of "marked depression and sedation." "Seizures" persisted at a fre-quency of 1–2 per month. The patient was referred for a pediatric neurology consulta- tion at an academic medical center, where it was felt that zonisamide might be of benefit. Levetiracetam was also considered but excluded due to the risk of psychiatric complications. Clonazepam was instituted but failed to control his anxiety. At age 16, he was being considered for a vagal nerve stimulator to control his "seizures." He was also being treated by his family with cannabinoids, their preferred treatment because it was "natural."

At about this time, my office location changed, and the parents decided to continue without neurologist involvement. This choice was discouraged by Barton's treating psychiatrist, but the parents never modified this decision.

Of note, the patient's severely impoverished social life was continuing unchanged. It was difficult to motivate him to interact with peers. He repeatedly said that he "preferred to stay home after school and on weekends and read books." He seemed to have little motivation to expend the effort or withstand the anxiety associated with making changes in his social and school life, explaining that his parents were "so controlling" that it was not worth trying. Every move he made would be "criticized," and new rules to "protect" him would be set.

During this period, Barton began treatment with a psychotherapist who supported Barton's growing desire to be free from his parents' unremitting control. To this point, virtually every attempt to set up an agenda for Barton's progressive treatment was countermanded by his parents. Also, during this time, he was brought to another neurologist for a second opinion. She concurred that it was impossible to determine what part of Barton's difficulty was biological and what part was psychological. Of interest is that Barton was personally able to observe and acknowledge the psychogenic features of his situation. However, his anxiety about engaging in a social life and opposing his parents blocked him from "taking chances."

During this period, Barton underwent a two-week comprehensive workup at a Southern California referral center. Their impression was consistent with that of his local physicians, and they made no recommendation about a change in medication. An interesting comment from his pediatrician at this point was that she felt "very sorry" for Barton, citing his family's control as a major factor in his making so little personal progress.

In summary, this patient presented a very complicated history of behavioral difficulties and seizure-like events. He was resistant to multiple anticonvulsants and not amenable to surgical treatment for seizures. No clear structural lesion was ever identified to explain his "seizures." These events also occurred in the context of profound personal developmental delay associated with social avoidance and months-long absences from school. Involved was also an alleged attention-deficit hyperactivity disorder presumably resistant to medication, and a generalized anxiety disorder paired with severe depression. Multiple medication trials were completed. All except zonisamide and cannabis were ineffective and zonisamide needed to be withdrawn because of anorexic side effects.

Central to this case is family pathology. Barton's parents had an unrelenting need to direct his treatment and, indeed, his life. To the extent that he developed a chronic socially paralytic condition, his "seizures," played into their need. Barton needed his parents and their approval, and for the most part could not effectively oppose their control over his life. He actually tried to grapple with them but was weak in his attempts. According to Barton, all attempts to extricate himself from his parents' control at first failed. In his words: "they wouldn't even let me even breathe without warning me that there is dust in the air and I could have an anaphylactic reaction."

But that wasn't the end of this story. At that point, at age 16.5, Barton entered into a new and radically different psychotherapy with a new psychiatrist-psychotherapist. His first move was to join the school swimming team. To everyone's surprise he not only liked the freedom of swimming and being part of a peer group but Barton was an excellent swimmer. At about the same time Barton became friendly with a "wild kid." The first time they tried to run off and drink together, but were caught. The punishment was an indefinite 7:00 P.M. curfew. But this time – aided by the support he received from his new friends and psychtherapist – Barton asserted himself and began an impassioned climb toward, as he put it, "real life."

Author's Comment:

Barton, in spite of his systemic illnesses, was irrepressible in insisting that he could and would become "normal." Sadly, at first, his parents' well meaning but stringent overprotection prevailed and he remained socially inhibited and overly cautious in virtually everything he attempted. It may be of interest that now, after his tirelessly working to overcome the barriers that prevented his progress, he is in college. His preformance is good and he is intending to beome a psychologist. Because of his alleged seizure disorder he cannot yet drive but he is determined otherwise to live a "normal' life, and indeed he is progressively achieving this.

Complexity Summary

1. Biological (including genetic)
   Acute:
   – History of severe atopic reactions in first years of life.
   Chronic:
   – Allergic susceptibility (dermatological, respiratory)
2. Psychiatric/psychological
   – Rule out ADHD, becoming overwhelmed in social situations (rule out social phobia), hypersensitivity to noise.
   – Rule out Tourette's syndrome, later overshadowed by tonic-clonic seizures, of undetermined etiology, lasting two years.
   – Hyperreactivity, so that virtually all physical and emotional provocations were seen as overwhelming if not traumatizing for Barton.

3. Social (including family and other support systems)
   - Parental control over virtually all aspects of patient's life holding to the "threat" that he was not safe existing on his own.
4. Care delivery, including access to care
   - Somewhat limited, for example, when I (Mendius) changed office locations and when the family could not retain a neurologist, they worked with for a year at UCSF they opted to go without one.
5. Fundamental factors supporting or obstructing the treatment, in particular quality and continuity of the physician–patient relationship
   - Barton was intellectually gifted and psychologically insightful, strengths that progressively came to the fore in support of Barton's progress.
   - Barton's parents closely regulated his treatment. To receive their full support treatment, Barton had to conform to their restrictions, even though their conscious motivation was protective. Barton later became more vocal about his need for independence, including support for making decisions on his own. In very small increments, Barton was beginning to have his way, in part supported by tight bond with his current psychiatrist–psychotherapist.
   - Surprisingly (paradoxically), the parents always supported the current psychiatric/psychotherapy treatment, as if they subliminally appreciated its centrality for Barton's ultimate health.

Chapter 13
Management of a Teenager with Anorexia Nervosa: a Family Medicine Perspective

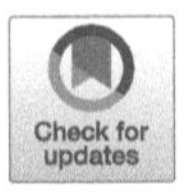

Elizabeth Etemad

A 14 year-old female, Molly, presented to our clinic in 2010. Concerns were restrictive diet, excessive exercise, recurrent injuries from competitive sports, rapid weight loss, lanugo, and the development of secondary amenorrhea. The onset of weight loss followed a break up with a boyfriend and placement of orthodontia. There was no evidence of bulimia nervosa or other purging behavior. Binge eating of a limited number of putatively "healthy" vegetable food sources (e.g., carrots and fruit) was noted. Menarche occurred without incident in 2008 at age 12.

The patient's mother identified concern about her daughter's weight loss prior to her first visit. The mother followed Molly's care closely and formed an alliance with me supporting her daughter's care. I discussed the options of counseling and referral to a psychiatrist for management of psychotropic medication. Nonetheless, the mother resisted having her daughter see a psychiatrist because she did not "want her daughter to be labeled." I was disappointed, but agreed instead to closely monitor her psychiatric and physical status during frequent visits for medical appointments.

Molly's anorexic phase started following pressure from a boyfriend to be sexually active before she was ready. Disappearance of secondary sexual characteristics can be brought on by a girl's reluctance to progress developmentally. Weight loss can cause amenorrhea, which lowers risk of fertility, reduces conventional attractiveness (smaller breasts, smaller buttocks, and lanugo), and "buys time" for a girl to be more advanced cognitively and emotionally before she is exposed or reexposed to sexual attention. Low estrogen and loss of menses can reduce emotional irritability and mood swings that normally occur with menses. As such, attempts to recommend oral contraceptive pills (OCPs) frequently meet with resistance by these patients. Girls know that there can be weight regain and breast enlargement associated with OCPs. OCPs prevent fertility, but would also reopen the door to

E. Etemad, DO (✉)
Family Medicine, Prima Medical Group, Novato, CA, USA
e-mail: eetemad@primamedgroup.com

© Springer International Publishing AG, part of Springer Nature 2018

S.A. Frankel, J.A. Bourgeois (eds.), *Integrated Care for Complex Patients*,
https://doi.org/10.1007/978-3-319-61214-0_13

being sexually active and force a girl to be more proactive with saying "no" to sex if she wishes to continue to abstain.

I also recommended that Molly have monthly osteopathic manual therapy (OMT) visits with me for her injuries related to her sports involvement. A comprehensive plan was implemented that included my following her weight closely, counseling about diet and exercise, and treating her with OMT while encouraging her to discuss in "free form" what bothered her at each visit. I offered her mother a referral to a psychiatrist later as well.

My recommendation for OMT was based on knowledge of how problematic the process of orthodontia placement can be for children and adolescents, and understanding that introduction of orthodontia at times may coincide with other stresses of emotional and physical development. My offer of OMT was in part based on my successful experience with another teenage patient several years earlier who had anorexia nervosa. I had studied cranial osteopathic manual techniques taught by a dentist who worked with the osteopathic community. These techniques help reduce jaw muscle dysfunction, dental discomfort, and reduce gag reflex triggered by placement of orthodontia. I learned of children and adults who were seriously compromised by the placement of orthodontic appliances that interfered with swallowing, as well as the accompanying dental pain and consequences of an impaired gag reflex. The following is a snapshot of Molly's character, her personal capacity for self-discipline being etiologically relevant to her evolving anorexia nervosa (Debra 2005).

Molly had never used drugs or alcohol recreationally. From the time of referral, she was, and continued to be, an excellent student; for example, she won a 2-week trip to Europe following a high school academic competition. During high school, she participated in multiple competitive sports including swimming, cycling, lacross, track and field, and softball. In 2012, she was an invited participant in a national cycling team competition, winning a scholarship from a sports equipment company. After high school graduation, she was admitted to several academically prestigious universities.

Molly's parents and brothers were also being seen in my medical practice. Both parents were college-educated and held professional positions outside of medicine. Two brothers were younger than her. Her family medical history included her mother with Raynaud's phenomenon, fibromyalgia, Hashimoto thyroiditis, sleep apnea, polycystic ovarian disease, allergic rhinitis, and asthma. Her father had gout, mild central obesity, and hyperlipidemia. One brother had ADHD and asthma, and the other allergic rhinitis.

Molly's past medical history was notable for multiple sports associated injuries dating since 2008 and included lumbar strains, chondromalacia patella, IT (iliotibial) band syndrome, patellar tendonitis, ulnar contusion with ulnar neuropathy after bike accident, MCL (medical cruciate ligament) sprain, hip flexor tendonitis, ACL sprain/synovitis, spondylolisthesis, loss of disc height at L5/S1 and L4/5 mild retrolisthesis, mild thoracolumbar scoliosis, scapular and rib pain from TOS (thoracic outlet syndrome), and an ovarian hemorrhagic cyst. A rheumatology consultation revealed Raynaud's phenomena, overuse injuries, and elevated CPK and AST due to muscle breakdown. There had been a 18-pound weight loss between 2008 and 2010, temporally associated with restrictive intake and excessive exercise.

Additional consultation included physical therapy between 2010 and 2013 to reinforce decreased volume of exercise, core abdominal strengthening, IT band and TOS stretches, and use of knee elastic neoprene braces. She was advised not "work through" pain, but instead cautiously build muscle. She had seen a chiropractor who claimed that he could "cure scoliosis." The patient continued with chiropractic care with my caution that chiropractic care was likely to help somatic dysfunction only.

When considering this background, ask yourself what might have driven this young woman to engage in this level of unrelenting physical activity? Adolescence is traditionally considered a time for interpersonal experimentation often in the form of rule-breaking activity. For this young girl, her deviation from the "norm" involved a dedication to challenges, leaving little room for age-appropriate "fun." Medical intervention was required repeatedly in part because of her frequent injuries.

To understand her recovery, make note of the support she received from me, her PCP. I have young children of my own and I enjoy working with teens as well. My goal was to provide her with a credible adult model for assisting in her recovery from AN as well as engaging her in a revision of her punishing lifestyle. The complexity of this case thus pivots not just on the association of AN and repeated orthopedic injuries, but also the irrationality of Molly's drive to succeed even while harming herself.

Details of Molly's descent into AN and her recovery are as follows. This process is presented using myriad, selected medical details taken from the patient's much more complete medical record. Beneath this barrage of detail was a young woman struggling to make sense out of her world and usefully deploy her talents.

At our first meeting, an 18 pound weight loss was noted (112 pounds, down from 130 pound). Lanugo (fine body hair associated with AN) was present. I received a telephone call from the patient's mother, concerned that her daughter was "yellow" after eating "lots of" carrots. Laboratory evaluation revealed elevated beta-carotene and BUN (27 mg/ml). Her CBC, blood chemistry panel, fecal occult blood, and liver function tests were within normal limits.

Over several sessions, Molly revealed she had been dating her first boyfriend who was 2 years older than she. In the context of this relationship, she felt pressured to be more active sexually than she found comfortable. After they broke up there was a time when she was not dating. Then she started a new relationship. Subsequently, Molly attended Planned Parenthood, and after two unsatisfactory trials of OCPs (oral contraceptive pills), which caused mood changes, she had a Mirena IUD placed. By that point she had experienced secondary amenorrhea for 8 months. At this time, she was participating in lacrosse, basketball, biking, and track. She complained of feeling lightheaded, with cold extremities, and fatigue. Weight was 118 pounds with BMI 19.2 kg/m2.

At a follow up visit, Molly's weight was 116 pounds. Her physical exam revealed lanugo, pallor, and sallow complexion. She complained of feeling faint with standing and this was associated with dizziness and palpitations. She was napping three times a day, experiencing hair loss, and had amenorrhea. The patient's mother reported that the patient was "snacking all day" on Power Bars. Her self-imposed diet consisted of a low carbohydrate diet otherwise. In the office 1 h after eating, her blood glucose was 79 mg/dl (low). It should not have been this low if she had eaten adequate calories. She was advised to complete a food diary for at least 2 weeks, get laboratory studies, to increase calories from carbohydrates and protein, continue to eat five meals a day, to increase water intake, and cut back her volume of exercise.

Still later in 2010, Molly's lanugo and amenorrhea persisted. She was less sallow and had a 5 pound weight gain to 121 pounds. Her mother reported that Molly was eating more. The patient's affect was better and she was more involved in our discussions than earlier. I again spoke to her mother about referral to a psychiatrist. Mother was reluctant, echoing her daughter's concern about being "labeled." As an alternative to psychiatric referral, I proposed treating Molly regularly with osteopathic manual treatment "for injuries and joint pain," recognizing the likely palliative (psychological) value of such a recommendation. I also told the patient's mother that regular visits could allow me to follow Molly closely and intervene if there was more weight loss. It is worth noting here that in primary care medicine, such "strategic" clinical moves are often necessary for engaging patients to follow an established treatment regimen and to stay away from counterproductive treatments.

Early in 2011, Molly confided that she had been feeling pressured to be sexually active and "almost had been." She had broken up with her (second) boyfriend a few months earlier (in 2010). She requested an OMT visit for neck, thoracic, and rib pain.

At a subsequent OMT visit, her weight was stable, menstrual cycles irregular, mood "good," although orthodontia was causing pain with eating. We continued manual therapy for facial, jaw, and neck muscle movement. I taught her a myofascial stylopharyngeus muscle technique to ease jaw opening and relieve spasm in hinges of the jaw (another example of the advantage of having a "kit bag" full of clinical tricks that will appeal to a patient, in this case an adolescent).

Later 2011: With mother's encouragement, Molly consulted with a chiropractor for recurrent somatic dysfunction. Mother was also worried about a thyroid disorder. Thyroid testing was normal. Molly also complained of low back and neck pain after weight lifting,

Still later in 2011: I learned that Molly had won a scholarship for a 2-week trip to Europe. Prior to Molly's visit, the patient's mother asked me to discuss safe sex with her. Consequently, I discussed with Molly when and how to negotiate sex, discussed safe sex with condoms and relevant privacy issues, and role-played managing demand for sex. Molly agreed to a trial of norethindrone/ethinyl estradiol OCP and to continue to use condoms when sexually active. The trial was discontinued by patient after several weeks because she felt "bloated."

Still later in 2011, she presented with diarrhea and right lower quadrant pain with rebound. GI laboratory tests were normal. She disclosed with mother out of room that an IUD had been placed the month before at Planned Parenthood. Urine pregnancy test was negative, chlamydia was negative, and stool for blood was negative. CT scan revealed a left ovarian cyst and no appendicitis. Ultrasound showed a hemorrhagic ovarian cyst. She completed antibiotic and antifungal therapy for group B streptococcus and yeast infection which were also identified. After this, she continued to have stool changes and abdominal cramping a month later. I discussed a referral for GI.

At her consultation with the GI specialist, the specialist did food allergy tests which were negative for dairy and wheat allergies.

She had adopted a vegan diet after viewing the movie "Forks Over Knives." We determined that she was eating too much quinoa and rice (six servings at a time). Her weight had decreased to 135 pounds from 138 pounds. I discussed with her that I was concerned that she needed to meet significant protein/calorie needs with her level of exercise. I recommended that she add back shellfish, fish, tofu, nuts, peanut butter, beans, eggs, and lean chicken/turkey.

At this point, in her senior year of high school, Molly's personal story began to take a more normative character. In 2011, she received a college scholarship from a national sports equipment company, having maintained a 4.0 grade point average throughout high school. She was happily dating a boy she met on the trip to Europe. She had plans to cycle at university on a competitive team.

Medically, she was less tumultuous. I recommended evaluation of prolactin, LH, FSH, DHEAS, and testosterone because her cycles were still irregular. Results were all normal except that FSH:LH were suppressed. Thyroid antibodies were negative. The Mirena IUD can cause amenorrhea which can necessitate lab testing if a clinician is concerned there is an eating disorder still present.

At a follow-up 2 years later, she was a engineering undergraduate major at a major Midwest university. She had stopped competitive cycling, but still swam an hour a day. She had another boyfriend who was respectful of her choices. She had gained weight (maximum 141 pounds). She was still using the IUD due to OCP's side effects. Menses were regular. She was doing well socially with no return to anorexia nervosa behaviors.

Commentary by Author

As a female physician, I wanted to develop an alliance with this patient with the objective of helping her negotiate the challenges to becoming a strong young woman, not afraid to pursue a challenging professional career, and able to resist unwanted social and sexual pressures. I also wanted her to have counseling about mental health issues as well as instruction about how to avoid injuries as an athlete, maintain good nutrition, and avoid unintentional pregnancy/STDs.

Frontal lobe development leading to reduced risk-taking and improved judgment lags behind physical maturity in both girls and boys (Johnson et al. 2009). Adults frequently mistake physical maturity for adequate social judgment. Teen boys frequently date younger teen girls who are not prepared to make decisions about their sexuality, as was true in this case. Girls are often under intense social pressure without having adequate skills or judgment. They may at the same time be afraid of, yet interested in, sexual relationships, ambivalence impeding their social decision-making capability.

Birth control counseling is frequently welcomed by these young women, but practically speaking birth control is a complex skill for girls to negotiate. The burden is mostly on the girl. Birth control does not work well for everyone. Condoms fail. Teens frequently do not know about the "day after pill." Contraceptive management is frequently sought after the first sexual encounter, but not before. Girls may experience practical barriers to acquiring and using birth control medication. These medications may make them feel unwell. They may be embarrassed about buying them. They may with good reason be afraid that their parents will see the medical bill for the chlamydia screen or contraceptive management. Then there are all the personal moral dilemmas. No wonder girls retreat and reconsider. Note also their professional future and financial health often depends upon delaying the first child and preserving fertility at the same time.

Complexity Summary

1. Biological (including genetic)
   Acute:
   – Molly's initial presentation was for physical complaints and a behavioral sequence leading to the diagnosis of anorexia nervosa (AN). Over time, other acute physical symptoms became manifest.
   Chronic:
   – The underlying chronic issue was anorexia nervosa, as discussed below. Molly remained chronically at risk for metabolic, cardiovascular, gastrointestinal, and musculoskeletal complications of AN, all of which required periodic surveillance.
2. Psychiatric/psychological
   – Anorexia nervosa has significant comorbid psychiatric risk of anxiety, mood, and personality disorders. A minority of patients become so unstable that they need inpatient care. Residential treatment, often for weeks or even months, may be required. Typically outpatient management involves ongoing psychiatric care and psychotherapy, as well as medications. Osteopathic manipulative medicine (OMM). This patient and her family were resistant to psychiatric referral; so, she was managed solely in a primary care model, emphasizing supportive understanding from her trusted PCP. With such management, surveillance for symptoms of instability that would require a prompt psychiatric referral (looking for psychosis, suicidality, <10% BMI, bradycardia <50 bpm, systolic blood pressure <90, orthostatic, temperature <96 F, arrythmia, syncope, potassium <3.2, serum chloride <88 mmol/L, intractable vomiting from esophageal tears, and failure to respond to active treatment) is needed (Rome et al. 2003).
3. Social (including family and other support systems)
   – This patient had adequate housing, social support, and medical insurance. Her family was available and attentive, mother interacting regularly with the PCP.

4. Care delivery, including access to care
   - She apparently had regular and ready access to her providers; in this case, primary care was delivered by a physician specializing in family medicine. She would have had access to psychiatric care had she accepted it. Ancillary supports such as Planned Parenthood were judiciously engaged.
5. Fundamental factors supporting or obstructing the treatment, in particular quality and continuity of the physician–patient relationship
   - Because this case involved systemic medical and psychiatric comorbidity, it represents a "medically complex" case. From a systems point of view, it is also "complex," as the PCP became a coordinating physician (Frankel and Bourgeois 2013), overseeing all medical and interpersonal management issues. In addition, as part of her clinical work the PCP chose to replicate the function of a psychiatrist–psychotherapist. An added strength of this successful case was the long-standing working relationship between parents and physicians, and the development of an analogous bond between patient and physician.
   - The potential seriousness of this case, with the risk of development into medical and psychiatric collapse, is masked by the strength and persistence of her PCP's clinical work.

References

1. Debra Katzman MD. Medical complications in adolescents with anorexia nervosa: a review of the literature. Int J Eat Disord. 2005;37(1):S52–9.
2. Johnson S, Blum R, Giedd J. Adolescent Maturity and the Brain. J Adolesc Health. 2009;45(3):216–21.
3. Rome ES, Ammerman S, Rosen DS, Keller RJ, Lock J, Mammel KA, O'Toole J, Rees JM, Sanders M, Sawyer SM, Schneider M, Sigel E, Silber T. AAP guidelines "Children and adolescents with eating disorders: the state of the art". Pediatrics. 2003;III:204–11.

Chapter 14
Man with Downhill Post-CVA Course Complicated by Loss of Wife's Support Due to Her Own Illness

Elizabeth Etemad

This was a case of a 68 year old man, acutely post cerebrovascular accident (CVA). Additional illnesses included cardiac dysfunction, diabetes mellitus (DM), macular degeneration, anemia from gastrointestinal bleeding, and depression. Patient's already complex medical care was seriously impaired from complications of a stroke and further compromised by loss of a spouse's assistance due to her diagnosis of a brain tumor. This case illustrates how Dr. Etemad efficiently used a home health nurse and closely tracked patient's health to manage this situation

Mr. B. was a 68 y/o businessman whose treatment course perfectly illustrates how integrated care and involvement of a registered nurse care coordinator (in this case from our Accountable Care Organization, i.e., ACO Medicare pilot plan) can be helpful, and at times critical, for managing a complex case.

As part of the current episode, in 2012, Mr. B sustained embolic strokes involving his occipital, temporal lobes, and cerebellum. He had a past medical history of dyslipidemia, congestive heart failure (CHF), renal insufficiency, and coronary artery bypass graft (CABG) with bare metal stents in place for coronary arterial disease. Other issues were iron deficiency anemia (not hemolysis since Coombs studies were negative), type 2 diabetes mellitus requiring insulin complicated by retinopathy and peripheral neuropathy, age-related "dry" macular degeneration, and previous cataract surgeries. He had normal vitamin B12 and folic acid levels. His HbA1C goal was shifted to less than 8% from 6.5% due to hypoglycemic episodes. He also had benign prostatic hypertrophy with nocturia causing awakening 2–3 episodes a night. He had repeated hospitalizations for complications from GI bleeding due to arteriovenous malformations in the intestines, diverticuli, history of ulcers due to *H. Pylori*, and recurrent colon polyps. He complained that he was taking a total of 18 pills a day. On formal count the total was actually 25.

E. Etemad, DO (✉)
Family Medicine, Prima Medical Group, Novato, CA, USA
e-mail: eetemad@primamedgroup.com

© Springer International Publishing AG, part of Springer Nature 2018
S.A. Frankel, J.A. Bourgeois (eds.), *Integrated Care for Complex Patients*,
https://doi.org/10.1007/978-3-319-61214-0_14

Mr. B. developed suicidal ideation in November 2012 without formal plans to harm himself. This development occurred 3 weeks after he stopped taking trazodone 50 mg at bedtime for sleep. trazodone had been prescribed for 10 months following his embolic strokes. His cardiologist suggested stopping it because he was concerned it was making him feel enervated and causing orthostatic hypotension. Taking into account his PHQ-9 (depression) score of 16 and Mini-Mental State Exam (cognition) score of 26/30, I resumed trazodone 50 mg at bedtime and added Escitalopram 5 mg in AM for mood and anxiety. Follow-up 3 weeks later revealed improved sleep and anxiety and a PHQ-9 score reduced to 8.

The history of the current illness is as follows. This unfortunate gentleman had a history of recurrent GI bleeding due to gastric ulcer from H pylori, arteriovenous malformations (AVMs) throughout his intestine as well as severe diverticulosis, and recurrent tubular colon polyps. In April 2012, his hemoglobin had dropped to 8 g/dL and he was transfused 3 days before. Just after this, his warfarin anticoagulation was held due to the active GI bleed. Then he presented with embolic strokes from atrial fibrillation. I followed him as an outpatient and addressed his suicidal ideation in November, 2012. He was maintained on medication for atrial fibrillation and anticoagulation. Despite these measures, in January 2013, he was found unconscious by his spouse at home and had seizures in the emergency department of the local hospital. He spent 3 days intubated in the ICU, initially in a coma. He was transferred from the ICU when alert and breathing well and then spent 5 more days in the hospital where levetiracetam was started. Once his breathing stabilized, he was sent for rehabilitation to a skilled nursing facility (SNF) for two weeks. He was maintained on levetiracetam in spite associated mood irritability and significant interference with memory.

Three weeks after discharge from the SNF, he presented with right lower lobe pneumonia from aspiration. He was treated as an outpatient. At that time, he was also referred to otolaryngology for a diagnosis of partial vocal cord paralysis resulting from prior intubation. His condition stabilized, gradually improving over 2 years. However, he was quite ataxic and suffered from visual neglect.

He was referred for outpatient neuropsychological testing that confirmed a memory deficit and received treatment at a neuro-rehabilitation hospital. He was eventually weaned off levetiracetam with little improvement in his ability to retain information. In April 2014, he came to see me for two visits and was discovered to have missed doses of furosemide, exacerbating his hypertension and early congestive heart failure. His congestive heart failure worsened and he gained seven pounds in 1 week. Daily rechecks in the office were instituted until his medication compliance improved.

I sent our ACO registered nurse to do a home assessment and she found another significant medication error. He was taking two anticoagulants at once. We decided to have the nurse set up his medication box and go to his home for monthly visits. We instructed Mr. B and his wife to do daily weight checks and call me with any indication of sudden retention of fluid. However, she was unreliable about communicating.

At first we attributed Mr. B's wife's lack of reliability to her preoccupation with running the family business in spite of her responsibility to care for her seriously disabled husband. Subsequently, his wife was discovered to have a large frontal lobe brain tumor, explaining her neglect. This created a new family crisis and the wife was hospitalized for brain surgery an hour away from home. I engaged the couple's children to help with caring for their cognitively impaired father. In spite of home care, in his wife's absence Mr. B skipped several doses of furosemide (a powerful diuretic) because he did not want to have incontinence. This triggered development of congestive heart failure and a potential hospitalization. I predicted this might happen and I asked him to see me that week for a check up. I was able to prevent hospitalization because I was quite familiar with his lifestyle and habits and instituted catch up doses and a mandatory stay at home one day.

Both the patient and his wife were cared for at home with full-time caregivers and a private geriatric RN case manager. Their children worked together to coordinate their parents' care. The ACO nurse visited monthly to try to prevent medication error (failure to get medication refills and take medication as prescribed) and prevent duplicate therapy given that there were multiple prescribing physicians. Two of his physicians, his cardiologist and myself (a family physician), are on the same electronic record and can view one another's medications. The endocrinologist, neurologist, and sleep apnea physicians were not on the same electronic record, but we asked them to inform us about medication changes so I could prescribe and monitor for side effects.

Mr. B died after his wife had the brain tumor resection. She had several strokes at the site of the tumor bed and lost all memory of her lengthly marriage. Her personality changed and she was disoriented. Following Mr. B's realization that she did not remember him, Mr. B. gave up hope and told his son he did not want heroics to save his life, requested enrollment in hospice, and passed away in hospice care within 2 weeks of stopping Furosemide, anticoagulation, and anti-arrythmics medication. Years later, his wife still does not remember that he died (though I know she adored him prior to the tumor surgery), but recently she has been doing much better than I would have expected. She has transitioned to a memory care skilled nursing facility and still works with her original private case manager.

Postscript: The decision to involve our group's input in our discussion of this case was very helpful. Our sleep apnea physician discussed side effects from escitalopram and risk of aggravating restless leg syndrome (RLS). Our neurologist/sleep specialist pointed out that after stroke there can be significant issues with central sleep apnea. In response, I weaned the escitalopram without difficulty, switched to melatonin 3 mg, and continued trazodone. Our patient's subsequent sleep study showed central obstructive sleep apnea. His cognition and mood improved with continuous positive airway pressure (CPAP). His sleep quality, RLS, and nocturia also improved. Of relevance to this case, CPAP for sleep apnea also lowers risk of atrial fibrillation and myocardial infarction.

Mr. B was taking daily iron supplementation, yet his iron stores were low due to continual slow GI blood loss. Another internist from our group recommended

                                                                E. Etemad

regular blood draws for hemoglobin and iron paired with outpatient 200 mg iron sucrose IV infusions at intervals to prevent need for transfusion. He was evaluated by the nephrologist and did not need erythropoietin to stimulate the production of red blood cells, as was originally thought.

Our critical care specialist who runs a neurorehabilitation hospital and our neurologist also discussed the need for integrated care for stroke patients. Though he did have a swallow study done at the hospital in 2013 that showed penetration, on discharge the family and he were not viligent with thickening foods and he had a subsequent aspiration pneumonia. At that time, continuing anticoagulation for atrial fibrillation in face of an active GI bleed was controversial, but later studies have supported continued use of anticoagulants in these cases to prevent embolic stroke and the need for transfusions. We decided that it might be better to have him take one of the newer agents for anticoagulation rather than the warfarin. We felt that he would be more prone to medication error if he continued warfarin. He was switched to twice daily dosing. It also became clear fairly rapidly that he was no longer able to manage his medical care and measures needed to be instituted to make sure that he could be stabilized with outside help.

Complexity Summary

1. Biological (including genetic)
   Acute:
   - His acute medical illness was CVA (cerebrovascular accident i.e. "stroke") with functional limitations requiring rehabilitation.
   Chronic:
   - His background and contributory illnesses included CAD with previous CABG (coronary artery disease with previous coronary artery grafting), DM (diabetes mellitus), anemia, and macular degeneration, colonic polyps, and gastrointestinal bleeding.
2. Psychiatric/psychological
   - Depression is very common, with an incidence of over 50% in the first year post-stroke depending on the anatomical location of the CVA lesion and the exact clinical study. With this patient and in any depression episode, suicidal ideation can occur requiring prompt psychopharmacologic intervention. An additional psychiatric complication associated with cerebrovascular disease and also notable in this case is vascular dementia. It can be acute or chronic, and often is present to some degree before a stroke and then can be worse after a stroke. Intervention with antidepressants (as in this case) is often associated with functional improvement. Caution needs to be used, as serotoninergic antidepressants should be avoided in the immediate post-CVA period with hemorrhagic stroke, as rebleed risk is problematic.

3. Social (including family and other support systems)
   - This patient's wife was distracted by the real-world work need to maintain the family business, compromising her ability/willingness to care for her husband. This development left him unsupervised which proved problematic when he could not manage his medications safely. During this period his wife, the primary caretaker, developed a brain tumor further complicating her husband's management despite the addition of in-home care support.
4. Care delivery, including access to care
   - Once mobilized, a comprehensive care team of several specialty providers (including physicians and nurses) was able to manage this man in a coordinated fashion. The coordination by the ACO nurse continued to be a critical and ongoing part of this patient's care. It appears that he had adequate access to insurance, medications, physicians, and other services.
5. Fundamental factors supporting or obstructing the treatment, in particular quality and continuity of the physician relationship
   - This physician was able to coordinate care with family, private RN case manager, ACO RN, children, spouses, and specialists thanks to her knowledge of the family's evolving needs.

Chapter 15
A Convoluted Treatment Odyssey of a Severely Drug-Addicted Bipolar Disorder Woman in Her Early 20s

Paul Gilbert Jr.

Linda was a 20-year-old single woman. Her plans for an exciting year abroad in Asia became instead a journey through Hell. While overseas on a student exchange program, she became engaged to a local man she barely knew. When that relationship collapsed, she then impulsively flew to Europe, disappearing into an extended period of chaos and drug abuse progressively involving a broad spectrum of recreational drugs from hallucinogens to opioids. When she ran out of money, she finally flew home to rejoin her parents.

Several months after this episode, the patient's parents urgently requested a psychiatric consultation for Linda since her behavior was becoming increasingly problematic for them. She agreed to meet with me under protest, and did so only to placate her parents. Having recently turned twenty, she insisted that "absolute privacy and confidentiality" would be the condition of our working together. So, from the start I was at a disadvantage, cut off from other sources of information that might inform my evaluation and forced to depend on the patient, likely an unreliable historian, for history.

Fortunately, the patient was compliant with medical testing, making it possible to determine whether she was in any kind of drug-induced metabolic crisis or had contracted a serious infection from her drug use. Prior to my first session with Linda, her father provided me with a capsule history. Linda was living at her parents' home but they were unable to set any limits on her comings and goings. She had begun working at a retail store but was in danger of losing that job because of her unreliability. Although her parents had cut off her access to their money, she earned just enough on her own to buy drugs.

She had suffered a major depression at age 16 when she had taken an overdose of acetaminophen and alcohol. She saw a social worker for psychotherapy and a

P. Gilbert Jr., MD (✉)
School of Medicine, University of California, San Francisco, CA, USA
e-mail: paulgilbertmd@gmail.com

psychiatrist for antidepressants, but stopped both treatments prematurely. "Everyone loved" Linda in high school because of her expansive and gregarious personality. She was often the life of parties until her behavior became too much for even her "edgy" friends—at times she would engage in tirades about philosophical matters that tried everyone's patience. In spite of Linda's volatility, she successfully completed high school and was accepted at a university but decided to defer enrollment for a year to work and travel overseas.

Linda was adopted. Since it was a blind adoption (family of origin information was not available), no one knew anything about her biological family history of psychiatric illness (including substance abuse). Her grandiosity, irritability, and periods of mood changes suggested that bipolar disorder should be a part of the differential diagnosis. An episode of major depression is often the first sign of what will later develop into bipolar disorder. Hypomanic and/or manic episodes are often experienced months or years after an episode of major depression has resolved, where upon a diagnosis of bipolar disorder is applied to the case. The importance of the missing psychiatric background information later became clear only later when Linda located her birth father.

Linda canceled and then rescheduled her first appointment, then arrived a half hour late for a subsequent appointment. This would become a familiar pattern of missed or abbreviated sessions. I soon found myself wondering how much good I was doing for her. I liked her and found her intelligent, intrigued by her childlike inquisitiveness. I enjoyed discussing her experiences with meditation and existential philosophy, but refrained from confronting her with the evident contradictions between her expressed wish to live a "pure, chemical-free" life without medication and her reckless drug use. I was trying to build a therapeutic alliance, reminding myself that the goal of every session with resistant adolescent patients is to get them to come back.

To develop a therapeutic alliance with Linda, I had to walk a fine line between acceptance and confrontation. I had to confront her extreme, at times provocative, behaviors but in a way that did not rob her of a sense of self-efficacy. Humor and irony were important as much in the tone as in the content of what I said to her.

Linda would agree to come to sessions as frequently as necessary to reassure her parents that she was getting at least minimal help. She was clear that she was not ready to stop using drugs. She had just begun, she said, to explore all of the possibilities of various natural and synthetic drugs. She mentioned almost casually that she was using heroin "most days" but methamphetamine "only every other day." Her closest friends were other substance abusers who had bounced in and out of substance abuse treatment programs. She barely managed to keep her job by relying upon the kindness and tolerance of her boss. She was still living with her family, but in almost daily conflict with them. Each night she would pretend to go to bed and then sneak out of the house after she knew her parents were asleep.

On most days, I received urgent calls, emails, and texts from Linda's parents daily telling me of the latest screaming fight over her drug use. I had to skirt the margin between confidentiality and my desire to protect Linda from harm. While saying she wanted me to assure "absolute confidentiality," she nevertheless seemed reassured when I told her that her father had sent me an email. At first her father limited his contacts to these emails but then we exchanged voicemails as he and I developed an alliance for dealing with her drug abuse. To my surprise and relief Linda approved of communications with her parents. It has often been my experience with her patients that adolescents and young adults are comforted by communications with concerned parents, even if they publically deny that that they are. They may overtly rebel to assert their independence but are reassured by expressions of love from their parents.

Highly intelligent and well-informed about the dangers of the drugs she was using, Linda convinced herself that she knew more about these drugs than did I. In spite of her protests, she was unable to stop using methamphetamine, heroin, and a seemingly random and reckless array of injectable substances. In her communications, she seemed to be saying "Stop me before I kill myself." My technical challenge was to treat her, an adult behaving like a younger adolescent, with a course of treatment that would inevitably require the resources of a dual diagnosis program. She was experiencing both bipolar disorder and substance use disorder.

My initial posture was directed at building a therapeutic alliance despite the chaos she maintained in her life. I repeatedly rescheduled missed appointments and confronted her with her denial and the contradictions between her stated goal of a lifestyle free of artificial substances and her almost daily plunges into drug experimentation. She wrote me long, sometimes eloquent, emails expanding upon her spiritual interests and adventures in meditation. I engaged her in digressive discussions of Eastern religions, seeking a connection with her and looking for opportunities to ground her in reality. It was obvious to me that Linda would not be able to recover from her addictions and depressive disorder without a residential treatment program. However, she resisted and defeated all efforts to rein her in forcing me to find less direct ways of incorporating her in our work.

Creating a therapeutic relationship with Linda occurred in fits and starts. Linda's father repeatedly reached out to me. At first these communications were one-sided. I listened to his concerns and offered little in response except for expressions of empathy. His advocacy, however, was implicitly welcomed by both Linda and me. His involvement actually assisted me in consolidating a reliable place in our effort, first as Linda's advocate and then as a mediator in "tough love" discussions about limits and consequences. Often, I feared that I had "stepped over a line" and that my statement or action might destroy my relationship with Linda. If I rolled my eyes or gasped in disbelief upon hearing the fabrications she told herself, I did so with humor. Personally, she and I both knew that she was terribly lost and completely alone as she rationalized her decision to continue to use drugs. Ironically each failed attempt to rein in her reckless substance abuse served ultimately to build a shared case for residential treatment. The process was anything but smooth, however. Her labile mood and the variable effects of combinations of drugs substantially impaired her judgment.

Linda's father became a critical ally in my work. He sent me frequent emails that I in turn shared with his daughter. Linda slowly allowed her concerns over privacy—really fears of losing her independence—to take a secondary position as she moved toward accepting the need for adult limit-setting. A steady flow of text messages and emails from Linda's father made the therapy into something of a family intervention.

Note that the kind of judgment called for in this case is actually typical for virtually all therapeutic relationships. Sustaining a working relationship by "playing along," not challenging the patient, while frequently called for in psychotherapy, is often also appropriate when engaging a resistant patient to comply with other medical treatments. It was my hope that the healthier aspects of Linda's personality would prevail over her self-destructive impulsivity.

Linda's father called me after Linda sent an email to her parents and to her three older sisters (who she referred to as "my family of intellectuals") describing the appeal of suicide. She couched this as concern about her drug-addicted boyfriend and his statements about suicide as an attractive escape from his own nightmarish situation. During this time of extreme crisis, Linda began to arrive at sessions late in an irritable and grandiose state of mind. She was sleeping little as she "couch surfed" with various friends from night to night. She rejected all prescribed medications in favor of "natural" remedies. In my opinion, natural supplements like omega-3 fatty acids might have been useful in stabilizing her mood had it not been for the destabilizing effects of her habitual use of another preferred natural "remedy," mescaline.

Using whatever therapeutic alliance I could muster, I insisted that Linda meet with her parents and me in a series of family sessions. This effort was critical for channeling her parents' evident panic into a practical plan of action focused on finding a recovery program that Linda would accept. It became increasingly clear that treatment in a dual diagnosis program was essential. Yet, we had little leverage beyond saying that we loved her, were worried about her, and saw her escalating drug use as putting her on a road to an early death.

While Linda rejected all substance abuse treatment programs, therapeutic progress was evident in a series of seminal emails she sent to me summarizing her life history and her attempts to find a sense of belonging within her adoptive family. She "couldn't compete with" her older siblings whose accomplishments had eclipsed her own. She became convinced that her "defective genes" inherited from her biological parents were the unseen cause of her problem. She felt damaged and not worth loving. As a deflection from herself, much of her effort was directed at persuading her boyfriend's estranged parents to do a better job of caring for him. She claimed that she couldn't ask for anything for herself from her own parents.

Five months into treatment, unable to rescue her boyfriend from his heroin use, she descended into even more extreme IV drug use. At this point, she could not even remember what drugs she had tried from day to day. Any substance suggested to her was the next thing to shoot up with including methamphetamine and DMT (N, N-dimethyltryptamine). She was increasingly exhausted and exhausted those around her. She descended into an episode of depression which, paradoxically, made her more compliant with treatment.

Throughout all of this chaos, Linda maintained a discernable therapeutic alliance with me. She came to sessions late, but if she missed a session she was willing to reschedule. As much as possible, I confronted the contradictions between her intent and her behavior. This approach was tentatively successful and she agreed to an assessment at a dual diagnosis program in Tucson. She was finally willing to give treatment the try we had hoped for. However, en route to Tucson with her parents, she apparently had a psychotic episode, fled at a gas stop, and called 911 saying that she was an adult whose parents had abused her and were now kidnapping her. On the return trip home with her parents, she was pressed to agree to fly to the Tuscon progam with an escort.

She entered the treatment program in Tucson but after little more than a week refused to continue. Withdrawing from the program, she agreed to transition to a SLE (sober living environment) near her parents' home. While there were doubts about the program succeeding, her parents and I desperately needed help for her and perservered. The SLE proved to be anything but a place of sobriety. Drugs were freely available. She never attended a single NA meeting (which had been a condition of her contract with the SLE). She visited her boyfriend, who was now in jail on a drug trafficking charge.

After several weeks, I arranged to meet with Linda at a coffee shop close to her SLE. She looked tired and disorganized admitting that the SLE was "a joke," but she refused to return to her Tucson treatment program. Yet she did agree to a psychological testing evaluation in order to have a more objective source of information about the nature of her problem. The psychometric assessment provided further evidence for a bipolar disorder and the need for medications to stabilize her. The psychologist and I met with Linda to interpret the results of testing and the recommendation of a dual diagnosis program where she would initiate a trial of medications.

Four months later, Linda agreed to return to her original residential treatment program. This time, after a struggle, the program psychiatrist and I persuaded her to try valproate to manage her bipolar disorder. The result was impressive. On therapeutic doses of valproate, her grandiosity and impulsivity rapidly diminished. Yet she fled from the program several times and was each time readmitted with new behavioral conditions. I worked closely with the treating psychologist to create a combination of personal support, group therapy, imposed limits, and ultimately medication (without which her mania would have undermined the treatment).

In retrospect I have only praise for the treatment program. On staff were a psychologist, a psychiatrist, and addictions counselors. Many residents were young addicts with whom Linda could identify. The staff had the necessary sophistication to understand that Linda could not be optimally treated without mood-stabilizing medication. And, most important, they had the patience to see her through numerous runaways.

Linda completed the residential program in four months, thereafter moving from the intensive program to a step down facility. She agreed to remain in the Tucson area to avoid problematic relationships with street people near her parents' home. Four years later, on follow-up, Linda was continuing to live in Tucson where she rode her bicycle to and from work at a restaurant. She was with a new boyfriend who was not a drug user. She remained on valproate and in regular psychiatric treatment.

                                                                P. Gilbert Jr.

Author's Reflections

Linda's case illustrates the importance of forbearance in the face of opposition from a drug-dependent young adult, particularly when her presentation is complicated by significant comorbid bipolar disorder. A strong alliance with the parents was critical in this case as was a working collaboration with the residential treatment facility before, during, and after referral.

Cases like this one are encountered by PCPs frequently. As in other of our cases, e.g., the girl with anorexia nervosa (Chap. 13), the dedication and continuity of care appears to be central to case success. The patient in both of these cases needed to be "dissuaded" from a self-destructive course of action and "faith in" the treating physician seemed to play a significant part in achieving this. The systemic medical-psychiatric complexity presented itself in a different order in each case. For the patient with anorexia nervosa, the PCP's trustworthiness was established through her medical expertise. In Linda's case, medical intervention was not possible until a "therapeutic relationship" with the psychiatrist was consolidated.

Linda could not have been treated successfully without the support of her parents, psychiatrist, psychologists, and substance abuse counselors. Collaboration occurred daily throughout the course of her residential program. Frequent monitoring of her physical health was an essential aspect of her treatment. Her use of IV drugs elevated the importance of this aspect of her treatment in order to minimize dangerous physical effects of one or another of her street drugs.

Complexity Summary

1. Biological (including genetic)
   Acute:
   - Beyond her severe psychiatric illness, the patient did not present with acute systemic medical illness. However, within a year, her drug use became the central biologically relevant pathogenic factor in her life.
   Chronic:
   - While not chronically medically ill, the patient was at risk for systemic complications of drug abuse, e.g., HIV, HCV, cellulitis, vascular and dental complications of amphetamine use, all of which required continued surveillance and much of which she resisted.
2. Psychiatric/psychological
   - This woman's extreme substance abuse, bipolar disorder (eventually responsive to valproate), and ongoing erratic behavior, possibly consistent with a comorbid borderline personality disorder, were a significant source of personal and family distress. Expanding the diagnostic picture, this case illustrates well how "psychiatric multimorbidity," in this case the combination of personality disorder, depressive or bipolar disorder, substance use disorder,

the possible traumatic effect of her adoptive mother's life threatening illness, and unresolved adoption issues can warrant reclassification of an "only psychiatric" patient to a "complex patient" case.

3. Social (including family and other support system)
   - Throughout high school, the patient functioned adequately using her both intellectual and social skills ("everyone loved Linda"). She came from a family of plentiful financial means and was given opportunities that could have obscured the extreme and unorthodox nature of her behavior. Nonetheless, her earlier reputation was distinguished by being unconventional and popular with peers and adults. It was not until after graduation and a trip to Asia that she distanced herself from her highly supportive family. It is tempting to attribute this departure from her previously more contained lifestyle to her progressive abuse of street drugs.
   - Additionally, as noted above, this patient was adopted, a background that could have provided the basis for a major personality distortion (identity crisis), especially during adolescence. Adoption-based crises in adolescence are often distinguished by impulsive and antisocial behavior. Further destabilizing for Linda may have been her mother's recently diagnosed life-threatening illness.
4. Care delivery, including access to care
   - Coming from a well-resourced family, she had adequate access to insurance, medical care, medications, and residential care when needed.
5. Fundamental factors supporting or obstructing the treatment, in particular, quality and continuity of the physician–patient relationship
   - The challenge of establishing and maintaining a therapeutic relationship with this complex patient was the critical variable in this case. Over time, the interpersonally robust therapy relationship provided the substrate upon which the patient's psychopathology could be effectively addressed. The possibility that her adoption and her mother's illness could have played an etiological role in her erratic behavior adds to the challenge of doing psychotherapy with this patient.
   - The tenacity and skill of her treating psychiatrist/psychotherapist were repeatedly tested by the dangerous circumstances in which the patient put herself.

Chapter 16
A Professionally Successful Man with the Midlife Onset of Severe Depression and Associated Suicidal Intent

Paul Gilbert Jr.

Just before the holiday season in 2009, Mr. O. a 55-year-old electrical engineer fell into a different state of mind. Although under consideration for promotion, he abruptly resigned his position, certain that he was about to be terminated. He had convinced himself that his work was inadequate although he had recently been awarded several patents. The reassurance of friends and colleagues was to no avail. He found himself a part-time position teaching at a community college, but over the next few months, financial pressures began to mount, and he became increasingly despondent and hopeless.

Midlife depression is often triggered by stress. Positive changes like a promotion creating anxiety about continued performance may be as stressful as negative changes like failure or loss. In fact, in Mr. O.'s case both were present, but the balance was toward a toxic relationship with his unit supervisor that silently contaminated his work environment. So, his fear that he would not secure promotion was not without some basis in reality.

In February 2010 Mr. O. saw his primary care physician who prescribed mirtazapine 15 mg at bedtime and quetiapine 25 mg bid. Accurately diagnosing an agitated depression, she referred Mr. O. to me for an urgent consultation. At our first session Mr. O. appeared exhausted, having slept little for weeks. He was eager to talk and recounted his confused state of mind at the time he quit his job. In retrospect he felt humiliated progressively realizing all that he had impulsively "thrown away."

Mr. O. told me he had immigrated to California from his native Denmark in part because he had discovered that sunshine helped to lift the pall of winter blues. However the academic pressures in an unfamiliar culture became increasingly intolerable for him. As a child growing up in a small town in the north of Scotland, he recalled episodes of "sadness for no particular reason." He "never enjoyed life as some people do." While he always had "close friends," he struggled with passive

P. Gilbert Jr., MD (✉)
School of Medicine, University of California, San Francisco, CA, USA
e-mail: pgilbertjr@gmail.com

© Springer International Publishing AG, part of Springer Nature 2018   119
S.A. Frankel, J.A. Bourgeois (eds.), *Integrated Care for Complex Patients*,
https://doi.org/10.1007/978-3-319-61214-0_16

suicidal wishes that were most pronounced during the winter. In recognition of his brilliance, he received a full scholarship to university where he excelled. It was there that he met his wife Ms. O. who would become his "rock," the source of stability in his life and his reason for living despite his deep pessimism.

Depression is often a family illness. While midlife clinical depression may present without a prior history of treatment, a careful history will often reveal the childhood origins of the cognitive triad of depressive cognition: underestimation of past successes, low self-esteem, and pessimism.

I was very concerned about Mr. O.'s instability. His hopelessness was palpable. I asked about suicidal thoughts. He admitted having such thoughts for many years but especially now. He didn't have a plan for suicide and had never attempted suicide in the past. However, now suicidal thinking was more present. Mr. O. began each morning with a sense of dread asking, "What the fuck am I supposed to do?" In retrospect, he pictured that he had "screwed up life for himself and for his family." His wife told me that Mr. O. "didn't think he suffered from depression, just stupidity." He resisted the idea that his prized intellect might be influenced by depression distorting his judgment. However, the abstract concept that he suffered from a cognitive triad of negative thoughts filtered by his depressed mood intrigued him. In particular, Mr. O. preferred the idea that his depression could be genetic and that it might resolve leaving his intellect intact.

Mr. O.'s family history revealed a pattern of midlife depressions afflicting family members. Both his father and grandfather had experienced what in retrospect were serious depressions. His father quit his job as a chemist, abandoned the family, and went to work in the Middle East where the change of place and sunny climate apparently helped his mood. Mr. O. had learned only recently that his paternal grandfather had committed suicide at age 42. That depression might be the result of genetics further appealed to Mr. O. because if his state of mind was biologically based, apart from it potentially being treatable, it would not be seen a sign of "character weakness." Ironically, he did not view his dependency on his wife's support similarly.

Mr. O. was clearly at high risk for suicide and I recommended hospitalization. He was terrified of a psychiatric hospitalization since it would involve being separated from his wife and pleaded with me to find an alternative. In response, his wife promised to supervise his day-to-day activities at home and monitor his medications. I agreed tentatively to initiate treatment with daily outpatient sessions combined with aggressive use of medications. I prescribed sertraline 50 mg bid, doubled his mirtazapine to 30 mg at bedtime, continued zolpidem-CR 12.5 mg at bedtime or sleep, and recommended light therapy and omega-3 fatty acid supplements. I saw Mr. O. daily, both individually and with his wife.

Initial phase of treatment: The initial phase of treatment was fraught with uncertainty. Mr. O. was not sleeping more than a few hours at a time. He was unable to function without the assistance of his wife. Had it not been for her constant presence hospitalization would certainly have been necessary. His initial Hamilton Depression Inventory (Ham-D) score, a measure of the depth of his depression, was a worrisome 45 (a score of 16 is "sufficiently depressed" to warrant inclusion in an antidepressant pharmaceutical trial). Zolpidem helped him get to sleep but he woke up in the middle of the night unable to return to sleep.

I collaborated frequently with his primary care physician both to review his medical history and medication sensitivities and to benefit from her long familiarity with the family. She was in agreement with the plan to keep this patient at home if at all possible knowing of his vulnerability to shame.

Improvement: Within days of my initiating medications, Mr. O. noted "remarkable improvement." He described it as a return to his more familiar pessimistic worldview. He recalled a fragment of a dream in which he was typing on a keyboard and awakened to find his fingers moving as if he was typing a report. He took this as a predictor of return to normality. Yes, he would be working again!

Interpersonal psychotherapy (excerpts follow): In this context Mr. O. said he was perplexed that people were still often attracted to him despite his dark, self-deprecating sense of humor. I suggested that perhaps they might see through his demeanor to his essential warmth and generosity. He seemed not to understand the intent of my comment. His response was consistent with his depressive devaluation of his self-worth. He claimed that he preferred a socially isolated existence emphasizing "thinking" and had found a way to make his philosophical bent of mind a profession. In response, I said that while I appreciated his solace in solitude, choosing this mode of being might not work as well for him when depressed. At such times he might need to be more connected to others.

Mr. O. liked to debate epistemology, rationalism, and empiricism. How do we know what we know? His attitude was fundamentally skeptical. He took this tack with respect to evidence-based medicine as well. How could I know that anything I recommended would help? While this stance might be viewed as resistance to treatment, it was I believe, also a demonstration of his intact intellect and his reemerging sense of agency for his life. For Mr. O, at these times, discussion with me was little more than a parlor game with topics ranging from Aquinas to the Greek philosophers, his curiosity wide-ranging.

Regarding medication, over the course of the first month of treatment, sertraline was introduced and progressively increased from 100 mg to 150 mg and then finally to 200 mg daily. In response, Mr. O.'s anxiety decreased and his mood lifted. Quetiapine 50 mg bid also helped with anxiety. Despite his initial improvement, Mr. O. had frequent "black episodes" during which he descended into terrifying fantasies that he and his family would soon be homeless and living in the streets. When I said that his mood shift was his "depression speaking" and that he would be wise to ignore these thoughts for the time being, he was somewhat reassured.

The intermittency of black moods is not unusual during the recovery phase from a major depression. It was critical for Mr. O. that he had his wife's constant, loving attention and frequent sessions of psychotherapy with me. Without such support I believe his suicidal potential would have been too great to sustain outpatient treatment. It was also necessary that I involve his primary care physician in the medical aspects of his management for monitoring his weight, diet, and cardiac status throughout the treatment.

Since the beginning of this episode of his depression, Mr. O. lost 20 pounds. His appetite was poor. Diurnal variation of attention was demoralizing to a man accustomed to boundless, focused intellectual energy. Suffering from insomnia, he was tired much of the day. Dextroamphetamine 5 mg twice daily helped to increase his alertness but also added to his anxiety. Careful titration was necessary. A course of bupropion XL increased from 150 mg to 300 mg daily proved most effective for both ameliorating his depression and increasing his focus and concentration. For a man who lived by his wits, focus was of critical importance. As his mood improved by fits and starts, watershed moments began to occur when, for example, he could again enjoy his wife's chicken pasta.

Progress: Mr. O. began to reconsider his career options. He said he didn't miss the office and his colleagues as much as he missed team work. He began to look for ways to return to work but in a minimally pressured environment. His wife said supportively that she might return to her financial career to help support the family. Each day it was she who encouraged him to get out of bed, have breakfast, and go out for a walk whether or not he wanted to. His spells of despair continued, but not as deeply or as often as earlier. At end of the first month of treatment, I was able to reduce the frequency of our sessions to twice weekly.

Two months into treatment Mr. O. announced that he felt he was "returning to normal." He could socialize with friends without anxiety. He discontinued quetiapine without an increase in anxiety. His weight increased dramatically, up to a point where it was beginning to become a concern. Mirtazapine was then discontinued and sertraline reduced to 150 mg daily. His Ham-D was now 1! Three months into treatment Mr. O. continued on sertraline 150 mg daily and zolpidem for sleep. We further reduced the frequency of sessions to weekly then every other week then monthly.

During winter months Mr. O. had light therapy added to his medication regimen of sertraline 100 mg daily, bupropion 300 mg daily, and zolpidem 10 mg at bedtime. Within the past year he has stopped zolpidem and substituted melatonin 10 mg at bedtime. We now meet every 3 months. If he drifts into depression, often first noted by his wife, he increases his sertraline and schedules an appointment with me. He avoids stressors at work, keeps to a moderate work schedule, and is resigned to remain on sertraline and bupropion as long as necessary.

Complexity Summary

1. Biological (including genetic)
   Acute:
   - Beyond his major depressive episode, the patient did not present with systemic illness. It is usual practice to consider and screen for systemic causes of depression symptoms, such as hypothyroidism. In any patient with a depression as profound as this one, medical complications involving poor self-care (e.g., poor sleep and nutrition) may complicate the case.

Chronic:
- When depression becomes chronic, the above considerations must be addressed in an ongoing way. If depression does not respond to conventional treatments including medication and psychotherapy, other systemic explanations, e.g., vascular, rheumatologic, and oncologic illness, must be considered.

2. Psychiatric/psychological
- This is a classic case of major depression with an indefinable experiential precipitant. It is notable for its midlife presentation in the context of professional and interpersonal challenges of that life phase. Such a setting is frequently associated with depression complicating narcissistic personality disorder, i.e., an adjustment to life easily upset by encountered limitations and disappointments. This patient's treatment included multiple medications, light therapy, and psychotherapy. Given the profundity of his presenting episode (a Ham-D score of 45 is extraordinarily high), acute psychiatric admission and ECT needed to be considered and held as options "in reserve" until he showed functional and symptomatic improvement.

3. Social (including family and other support systems)
- The patient was professionally employed, well insured, housed, and well resourced and had stable intimate relationships with his wife and children. Having these personal resources supported the possibility of outpatient management of this case of severed depression.

4. Care delivery, including access to care
- The patient had adequate access to insurance, medications, and professional services. At one point, for example, he needed to see his psychiatrist on a daily basis.

5. Fundamental factors supporting or obstructing the treatment, in particular quality and continuity of the physician-patient relationship
- With the unceasing support of his wife, the patient was able to accept and begin to personally combat his illness. After an initial "flight into health" and subsequent relapse into depression, he assisted attempts to treat and became engaged and compliant with care. All this progress was facilitated by an excellent patient/physician alliance. No doubt, this working alliance allowed for improvement in his clinical status without his having to rely on high resource intensive interventions such as inpatient psychiatry, partial hospitalization, TMS, or ECT.
- It is important to understand the place of his wife in facilitating and guiding his treatment, as well as the place of his psychiatrist in respecting this need and understanding its centrality to the case.

Chapter 17
Escalating, Interrelated Systemic Medical and Psychiatric Illnesses with Unrelenting Suicidality

Catharine Clark-Sayles

Treatment between ages 60 and 81 of a woman with severe esophagitis and worsening spinal pathology, as well multiple other "experienced" (but not proven) maladies requiring ED attention. Alienation of her three children and other supporting people, as well as exhaustion of financial resources, resulted in repeated loss of health system resources. She received repeated psychiatric treatments, including periods of inpatient treatment that included ECT, but with little improvement. Of note are her attempts to reengage family through escalation of her psychiatric complaints including threats of suicide. Of clear benefit was the committed effort of her PCP, and repeated involvement of caregivers.

Mrs. Tanjier was a patient seeing an internist in our primary care medical group when I first met her in 1990 when she was 60. At that time her major complaints were "depression and back pain."

She reported a life-long history of severe depression beginning in a difficult childhood. Her father was an alcoholic and her mother had schizophrenia. She suffered physical, verbal, and sexual abuse. She seldom talked about her childhood, beyond glancing references to it as a "painful time," and typically followed by an abrupt change of subject or a comment like "I'm joking." She completed high school, worked briefly in retail, then married in her mid 20s "because of pregnancy." She and her husband had three children, two daughters, and a son whose place in her life is minimized as she tells her life story. What one hears instead is how she and her husband travelled and took classes in painting.

Mrs. Tanjier began psychotherapy at age 30 after being treated with ECT in her twenties and twice afterwards. She was a heavy drinker in her 20s and 30s, although she denied ever being "an alcoholic." She was hospitalized briefly after suicidal gestures in her 30s and 40s and received therapy from several psychiatrists. She again underwent six sessions of ECT in 1989 for intractable depression following

C. Clark-Sayles, MD, FACP (✉)
Internal Medicine, Geriatrics, Greenbrae, CA, USA
e-mail: clarksc@maringeneral.org

© Springer International Publishing AG, part of Springer Nature 2018
S.A. Frankel, J.A. Bourgeois (eds.), *Integrated Care for Complex Patients*,
https://doi.org/10.1007/978-3-319-61214-0_17

divorce from her husband. In 1990, when I began to treat her, she carried the diagnosis of chronic major depression and passive/dependent personality disorder. At that time, she was under the medical care of Dr. B and was being treated with phenelzine (a MAOI antidepressant). She was enrolled in an outpatient psychiatry program, attending 3 days a week for intermittent periods through 1995. From 1990 to 1992, she was tried on bupropion, trazodone, sertraline, and lithium in varying combinations. She did not drink alcohol at that time.

In 1990, she was 5′4″ tall and weighed 138 pounds. She began to have lower back pain radiating into her legs with weakness and numbness in her legs. Mrs. Tanjier underwent a laminectomy and fusion at two lumbar levels at age 64. Postoperatively she showed initial improvement but by 1992 was again reporting numbness and sciatic pain in her right leg and underwent an additional level laminectomy and removal of hardware from the prior surgery. She improved for about a year but then began to have severe pain with numbness and weakness in her legs. She began taking opiates for pain control several times a day. These were initially acetaminophen with codeine and later acetaminophen with hydrocodone.

Her depression worsened and a trial of sertraline caused intense side effects including headaches and nausea and was ultimately stopped. Lithium was weaned and discontinued. She subsequently tried several other antidepressants and anxiolytics. In 1994, with a new psychiatrist (Dr. Z.), she started (ludiomil, a tetracyclic antidepressant) and then added fluvoxamine and alprazolam. He encouraged her to get a pet and a roommate and to take classes at a nearby community college. She had her own home and endured several roommates who would initially be "wonderful" and then would either leave or become "problematic." Although she was largely estranged from her children, she expected them to find roommates for her and to help her with money for dental work. One daughter lived in a nearby town. Her son rarely spoke to her and lived about a four-hour drive away. Her youngest daughter and grandson lived in Oregon, about a one-day drive away, and also would visit on holidays. Typically, her depression would worsen around holidays and when her ex-husband would host their children for parties, cruises, and other vacations, including his new wife but excluding her.

As you read on, notice the "family therapy" side of the PCPs responsibility in this and similar cases, the requirement that the PCP understand the family's influence in aiding or exacerbating the patient's presenting medical problems. Systemic medical illness typically becomes the partial or complete responsibly of family members as parents age or regress. If the relationships are ambivalent the patient's medical condition can become exaggerated. As in this case, the patient may engage in a manipulative attempt to force the disinterested family members into greater participation in their care and support.

I began seeing Mrs. Tanjier more regularly in 1994 and initially focused mainly on her back pain. Many of these appointments were only partially symptom-driven and were largely for rendering personal support. Her neurosurgeon felt there were no remaining surgical options. Several referrals for outpatient physical therapy were not successful due to frequently missed appointments. Although she had once enjoyed swimming, she refused water therapy because she felt she was no longer attractive in a bathing suit. Later, she developed cataracts and was advised to have surgery. She was ambivalent about surgery, scheduling, and cancelling several times until having surgery in 1997 after she failed her driving exam and lost her license.

Note that the patient's intermittent sense of desperation and the way her impatience defeated well intentioned treatment efforts. She was erratic and in fact infantile, but she also was self determined and stubborn. She seemed to lack empathy, undermining the will of the most well meaning potential ally. At the same time, she was colorful and in some ways intriguing. It is a mystery that she kept going, kept finding champions, for as long as she did. This "survival" instinct is often not mentioned or fully appreciated when we represent cases like this with the balance of their co-morbid pathology toward the psychiatric.

Mrs. Tanjier often called the Suicide Prevention hotline or the local crisis center and occasionally during medical appointments stated that she needed to be hospitalized since she was "feeling suicidal." Often she would start her appointment dramatically by saying "I think I am going to kill myself" and then produce a big grin. I found this behavior difficult to interpret and when I asked her if suicide was a serious possibility, she would either claim to be joking or change the subject. When I contacted Dr. Z, he told me this was a common presentation and that he felt hospitalization would not be beneficial. Mrs. Tanjier went to the emergency department (ED, a term synonymous with emergency room i.e. ER) once or twice a year during the late 1990s complaining of depression or suicidal feelings. She usually was released home. In 1995, things got worse and she required psychiatric hospitalization. When she was discharged her depression worsened and required further intensive psychiatric attention.

In 1994, she began having increasing leg pain with walking. She was constantly fatigued, sleeping 12 hours a day. She began to complain of a lump in her throat and pain in her chest. Her appetite was poor, but she had not lost weight and was at 149 pounds by the end of 1996 (an increase of 11 pounds). An evaluation showed an enormous hiatal hernia with very poor esophageal motility. She began taking omeprazole to control her "heartburn" and investigating surgery for the hiatal hernia. She presented frequently at the emergency department with complaints of nausea, nervousness, and depression. In 1997, she underwent a Nissen fundoplication for her hiatal hernia but continued to have complaints of difficulty swallowing and sore throat.

Her leg pains were increasing with constant numbness in her right leg and pain in her left leg and she complained that she was "walking like a duck." In an attempt to determine if this was vascular or neurogenic claudication, she was scheduled for an arteriogram in 1998. It was cancelled by an episode of supraventricular tachycardia resulting in hospitalization and a cardiac workup. She had normal cardiac nuclear stress test but episodic atrial fibrillation/flutter. Digoxin was added to her medications and she began to use low-dose aspirin.

A spinal MRI (magnetic resonance imaging) demonstrated severe multilevel stenosis. An epidural cortisone injection encountered marked scarring and caused a prolonged spinal headache with leg pain relief for only about 10 days. After her negative experience with the epidural injection, she refused further invasive procedures. She was angry with her previous neurosurgeon and missed a series of appointments with him. He eventually refused to schedule further appointments and advised her to attend a pain management program. She continued on intermittent codeine and COX2 inhibitors but had an episode of hematemesis in 1999 and endoscopy showed the she had severe erosive esophagitis and breakdown of the fundoplication with a hiatal hernia extending nearly to the base of her throat. The NSAIDs and COX2 inhibitors were now contraindicated for pain. Instead, she was tried on gabapentin and a TENS unit. This provided some relief of pain and I referred her for outpatient pain management. As an aside, in 2000 she had Thanksgiving with her daughter, took a new roommate and, ironically was looking about as well as I had ever seen her. This kind of contrast, her appearance flamboyant and her medical condition dire, was repeated regularly during my experience with her.

In 2000, there were several ER visits for slurred speech and confusion. She continued to complain of inadequate pain relief and admitted to unilaterally increasing doses of her opiates and alprazolam. Dr. Z. continued to feel that inpatient psychiatric hospitalization would increase her dependency issues and that it was contraindicated. She began to attend another psychiatric partial hospitalization program several days a week but complained about being around "old people." Attendance was spotty. She reported that a "retired doctor friend" was pressuring her for her pain meds and money and I made an Adult Protective Services referral. In mid-2002, she arrived at my office with a friend asking for hospital admission, her bags were packed and she was admitted to the psychiatry unit. Further ECT was discussed and she refused. A social worker case manager started working with her as well as the social worker for the partial program.

During this period, she intermittently hired an aide for 1 or 2 days a week and engaged a financial planner to take over bill paying. However, Mrs. Tanjier was running out of money and clearly needed more advisory help. Many of her caregivers suggested that she move to an assisted living facility. She reported that Dr. Z was telling her to stay in her home and to get a new tenant. Her daughter was completely estranged and refused to help her find a new tenant. Mrs. Tanjier initially agreed to look at several facilities but after 6 months had not done this. When she did look at a few, she was horrified by "all the old people" she found. She was now 76, concerned about her appearance and occasionally asked about onabotulinumtoxinA (botox) "for wrinkles."

She had episodes of paroxysmal atrial fibrillation but because of her esophageal bleeding, occasional falls, and noncompliance with medicines she was not placed on warfarin. The absence of anticoagulation increased her risk of small strokes and vascular dementia.

She otherwise was doing well and in 2001 was discharged from the partial hospital program with a hired aide who took her for an outing 2 days a week. The aide did not work out because she was "patronizing." At about this time, Mrs. Tanjier reported increasing pain and was started on a fentanyl patch every 72 hours. With a lot of encouragement, she began doing regular pilates-based physical therapy and reported improved pain control, strength, and balance. After another roommate left, she became more depressed. She started back in psychiatric partial hospitalization program in 2001. Her social worker wrote a letter expressing concern about her use of pain medication after witnessing some episodes of over-sedation. Mrs. Tanjier began having fights with the financial advisor about her over-spending. He was pushing her to sell her home and move to assisted living. She was hospitalized early in 2002 after taking an overdose of alprazolam (taking 12 of the available 20 0.5 mg pills).

In 2002, after her social worker reported that she had been in bed for 2 weeks and had only eaten a small amount of watermelon daily, she was again admitted to the general hospital. Her esophageal evaluation showed a huge hiatal hernia with very poor motility. Gastroenterology said, however, that she was able to swallow but needed extra time to ingest food and liquid supplements to boost calories. While in the hospital she was eating well without complaints of being unable to swallow and all of us, including Mrs. Tanjier felt that the only other option—a PEG (Percutaneous Endoscopic Gastrostomy) feeding tube—was not desirable.

In early 2003, she had several episodes of slurred speech and some transient facial asymmetry was reported by a nurse during one of them. She then was started on warfarin but hated the bruises. She continued seeing Dr. Z. monthly. He felt that medication changes were not going to be helpful and she would respond best to social support and a pet. She saw a few interns from community mental health support services but this was erratic. Christmas 2003 saw worsening depression. This time she "hated the inpatient psychiatry unit" and refused to return to Senior Partial Hospitalization Care. She began running out of medication and presented to my office in opiate withdrawal. Her weight dropped to 126 pounds as she also reported having difficulty finding anything she wanted or could eat. She was hospitalized again with rapid heartbeat and an attempt to find an inpatient psychiatric unit to take her in transfer was unsuccessful.

By the end of the year she was again suicidal, very depressed, and losing weight. She began missing appointments with Dr. Z. He did not want to re-admit her to the psychiatric unit. She continued with an aide several days a week who would take her out shopping and to restaurants but when the aide left for a month in early 2005, she deteriorated. During visits, she would talk in a childlike voice and several times appeared overly sedated. She admitted to taking extra alprazolam and pain pills. She was re-admitted to the Senior Partial Hospitalization care program but often missed her van pick up. Checking her medication profile turned up some duplicate prescriptions for sedatives and opioids received during ED visits. She also had apparent noncompliance with her antidepressant for several months. At about this time, Ms. X ran out of money and her caregiver left. Mrs. Tanjier sold her house and moved to an assisted living facility. She was then able to have an aide again 2 days a week. Her caregiver returned and she was suddenly cheerful and oriented.

This event illustrates a sad fact about our health care system. Running out of money often results in restrictions of involvement by valued care givers. While Mrs. Tanjier was erratic and often noncompliant in her treatments, she consistently brightened up when a valued care giver re-emerged. Making this situation more difficult is that apart from myself and Dr. Z there were no people remaining in her life who were consistently committed to her. She had "burned them all out." But desperately needed them to care about her.

Ms. Tangier progressively developed bizarre eating habits, eating a single food for weeks at a time (e.g., crab salad or whipped cream). Often she would only eat if her aide brought food to her. She had worried about being "too fat" as her weight dropped to 112 pounds. In 2005, she was evicted for continuing to smoke in her apartment. She started a fire in a wastebasket with a discarded cigarette. She moved to another facility further north. She initially disliked it and "the old people" but did begin to decorate her patio and made a couple of friends. She began missing appointments with Dr. Z and reporting that he would not return her calls. Consistently he also did not return my calls. Her social worker and I again looked at inpatient psychiatric units and new psychiatrists but were unable to locate any. We ultimately found a psychologist Dr. K who began seeing her for psychotherapy but was unable to prescribe medications. Because she now lived further away from my office and did not drive she began having more trouble keeping appointments with me.

Ms. Tangier remained relatively stable but missed appointments at my office, using the ER frequently for "anxiety." This ER was at a hospital where I did not have privileges and I often did not get notification of her visits there. The doctor there gave her extra opioids and sedatives making it difficult for me to track compliance. Medical staff at her assisted living facility also worried that they were not able to adequately manage her medication. She was hospitalized for dehydration in 2008 with a weight of 98 pounds. In the hospital, she began eating and drinking almost at once and repeat evaluation of esophagus showed little change. The option of a feeding tube was again considered and discarded. Mild cognitive impairment with poor short-term memory and some decline in MMSE (mini mental status cognitive examination) performance was noted. The Senior Partial Hospitalization Program was not willing to reenroll her. She saw a psychiatrist for consultation about medications and he suggested a trial of thyroid supplementation which did not improve her depression and may have made her tachycardia worse. He did not accept Medicare and ongoing care with him was too expensive to continue on a self-pay basis.

In 2008, her apartment facility did substantial remodeling and she was temporarily moved out of her apartment. When she returned her cherished patio garden had been destroyed. She still had her dog and an aide visited 2 days a week, but there was little else that was dear to her remaining. She predictably deteriorated around holidays and whenever her aide left, making more frequent trips to the ED for "anxiety" or "depression." She often called 911 to be transported by ambulance to the ED. After a few hours, a sack lunch, and an extra alprazolam, she was sent home by taxi without hospital admission. Under Medicare rules, most of these ambulance trips were not covered and were billed to her. Her weight fluctuated between 100–108 pounds. She reported more fatigue and had some falls. She usually slept from 3 AM until 1 PM and spent more time in her room. We discussed enrolling her in hospice care but she did not have a qualifying "terminal" diagnosis. She was now in closer touch with her children but they expressed concern that frequent ambulance trips and aides were causing her to use up her money. She continued to smoke and was having more trouble with dyspnea and chronic productive cough. In 2009, she developed pneumonia and was hospitalized. A home for the aged residential facility agreed to take her on their inpatient geropsychiatry unit and she went there for a month. She was showing increased signs of dementia manifested by worsening short-term memory and MMSE scores.

She went back to her assisted living facility without much having changed diagnostically. She was continued on same medications with the addition of mirtazapine 45 mg at bedtime. She continued seeing the psychologist Dr. K and myself regularly. She also continued frequent trips to the ED. In a 3-month period, there were 7 ED trips. The owner of the assisted living facility had contacted her family asking that she be moved to a skilled nursing facility. The more distant daughter had her transferred to a local SNF without letting me know. The medical director of the facility took over her care, an event which is increasingly common and illustrates the increasing fragmentation of care across the spectrum of home/hospital/office and skilled nursing facility. She was at the new nursing facility for a few weeks when she called 911 complaining of pain and demanding to be taken to the emergency department at my hospital. From there she was admitted for a UTI (urinary tract infection) and adjustment of pain medications. She was then transferred to a different SNF (skilled nursing facility), but under my care. She was angry and depressed and missed her dog. She was in a shared room with another resident. She had stopped smoking by then but continued to eat poorly. The family hired a geropsychiatrist to evaluate her (again without talking to me); this physician suggested switching alprazolam to lorazepam.

During this final period in 2011, Mrs. Tanjier developed a fondness for several fashion-related reality TV shows often referring to the personalities on the shows as if they were intimate friends. She liked to sit in the courtyard garden of the assisted living facility remaining heavily tanned. Her local son-in-law visited weekly, her distant daughter visited about every 4 months. They requested a hospice referral, but hospice initially refused to accept her. Two months later, when her weight had dropped to 90 pounds, the hospice program agreed to enroll her. Hospice nurses visited her several times a month. Chaplains and a psychologist also saw her weekly. One prior hired aide visited occasionally. She remained much the same until developing pneumonia in late 2011 when she died.

Summary by Author Regarding Case Complexity

This case presented numerous challenges associated with different types (e.g., biological and psychological) and levels (e.g., accompanying management difficulties) of complexity. Mrs. Tanjier had long-standing depression and abrasive behavior both of which were resistant to many treatments, psychotherapeutic, and somatic. Her personality caused her to interact with family and caregivers in ways which pushed them away, even while demanding more care from them. By her report, family visits deteriorated in response to her complaining about not being sufficiently included and she often made critical comments about family and caregivers. These comments often were about others' appearance and diet. In day treatment programs, her attendance was so poor that she was typically asked to leave the program. Persistent smoking in her apartment resulted in her being evicted from one assisted living complex. She avoided socializing in her assisted living complex because elderly residents were "repulsive" to her. She did best with intensive 1:1 social support but cost and availability frequently became a problem. Challenges to coordination of care among distant family and a rotating cast of local caregivers and social workers frequently fragmented her care. Additionally, the physical move to a living arrangement distant from her usual medical care added to the disruptions in her care. Her ability to call 911 and be taken to the ED for episodes of emotional dysregulation resulted in a rapid depletion of her financial resources and poor medication compliance. Lack of available psychiatric resources created anxiety in her caregivers, my office staff and me, especially in the face of her often stated suicidal intentions. Pain management for her back was often difficult and her lack of motivation impaired her participation in physical therapy and pain management programs. Her swallowing difficulties, associated with her very poor esophageal motility, were real, and it was often hard to determine if her periods of weight loss were primarily due to depression and/or dysphagia from esophagus malfunction. Her bizarre eating habits and intense focus on weight lead me to believe in retrospect that she had a component of anorexia nervosa.

Complexity Summary

1. Biological (including genetic)
   Acute:
   – At age 64, Mrs. Tanjier underwent a laminectomy and fusion at two lumbar level vertebrae for lower back pain radiating into her legs and associated weakness and numbness. Postoperatively, she had initial improvement but by 1992 was again experiencing numbness and sciatic pain in her right leg, necessitating an additional level laminectomy and removal of hardware from the prior surgery.
   Chronic:
   – Dysphagia: Her swallowing difficulties, associated with her very poor esophageal motility, were real and it was often hard to determine if her periods of weight loss were primarily due to depression and/or dysphagia from esophagus malfunction.
   – Continuation of lower back pain: Her neurosurgeon ultimately felt there were no remaining surgical options.
2. Psychiatric/psychological
   – In spite of the patient's medical illnesses, this was consistently a psychiatric case with patient fitting the image of a "help rejecting complainer." Little ultimately satisfied her. See above summary for the numerous situations to which this description applies. Diagnostically this seems to be a case of com-

mingled borderline personality disorder with elements of anorexia nervosa, although the borderline personality disorder is clearly the dominant problem. Evidence to support this position includes the chaotic developmental history, relational dysfunction, substance abuse, somatization behavior, passive-aggressive approach to her own care (sabotaging helpful interventions), expecting the adult children to solve the problems that she created, demeaning comments and blaming of other.

3. Social (including family and other support systems)
   - The patient alienated all members of her family including her children. Personal attention was critical for her maintenance, and when a steady care taker could be employed she was likely to respond and feel supported. But this kind of resource was not always available.
   - Toward the end of her treatment (and life), her financial resources ran out, restricting the care that could be purchased for her, including individual care takers.

4. Care delivery, including access to care
   - This case illustrates the consequence of poor adherence to medical care, and the indiscriminate use of ED care and ambulance transportation. While her access to care was usually adequate, at least until close to the end of her life, she chose to use the ED for much of her "urgent" care, a very expensive habit indeed.

5. Fundamental factors supporting or obstructing the treatment, in particular quality and continuity of the physician–patient relationship
   - The formula in these kinds of treatments seems to have significantly to do with physician commitment and caring. Whatever the contribution from Mrs. Tanjier in encouraging that relationship, her PCP offered unconditional care right up to the end. Successful, ongoing personal and medical management in this case likely occurred primarily through that vehicle. We have seen this principle demonstrated in our illustrative cases repeatedly. Many of us chose to practice semi-independently (in the community) since it gives us the best opportunity for creating and maintaining a strong, ongoing physician–patient relationship.

Chapter 18
Severe Anorexia Nervosa Requiring Hospitalization and Parenteral Feeding: Ethical and Legal Complications

David Palestrant

This is a case of severe malnutrition due to anorexia nervosa. The clinical picture was extensively complicated by diminished capacity to make medical decisions due to delusional thinking. There was little family support and eventually none when a sister, the only original contributing family member, resigned from the case. Complexity in case management was elevated over time because of inability to obtain insurance coverage to treat the anorexia nervosa. Finally, there was conflict between the attending hospitalist and, myself, internist, neuro-interventionist, about the placement of NG (nasogastric) tube. Resistance to its placement created a life-threatening situation for the patient that necessitated intervention of hospital bioethics committee.

Definition of "decisional capacity": The ability, capability, or fitness to do something; a legal right, power, or competency to perform some act. An ability to comprehend both the nature and consequences of one's acts. "Capacity" relates to soundness of mind and to an intelligent understanding and perception of one's actions. It is the power either to create or to enter into a legal relation under the same conditions or circumstances as a person of sound mind or normal intelligence would have the power to create or to enter.

This is a highly complex case of a middle-aged woman with medical complications of anorexia nervosa and a complex medical presentation. Often, patients afflicted with this illness are younger. Middle-aged and older patients (most cases are women) are particularly prone to have poor clinical outcomes, not the least of which are due to the other psychiatric comorbidity common in these patients. This comorbidity may include substance use disorder, depressive and anxiety disorders, as well as psychotic disorders, delirium, and dementia due to chronic nutritional

D. Palestrant, MD (✉)
Neurology Critical Care, Kentfield Long Term Acute Care Hospital,
1125 Sir Francis Drake Blvd, Kentfield, 94904 CA, USA

© Springer International Publishing AG, part of Springer Nature 2018

S.A. Frankel, J.A. Bourgeois (eds.), *Integrated Care for Complex Patients*,
https://doi.org/10.1007/978-3-319-61214-0_18

deficiencies. Notably present in this case was the patient's nonadherence to treatment, including rejection of lifesaving medical interventions, requiring a formal declaration of diminished decisional capacity to implement. This admittedly complex situation was made more complex by significant disagreements among treating physicians about how to proceed in managing a decisionally incapable patient and the eventual withdrawal from the case by the only available family surrogate decision-maker. The integration of multiple specialists (as well as many other health care personnel) in managing this case is presented in detail, with all the challenges of forging a unified front for the care of such an unfortunate, complicated, and trying case.

Ms. Y, at age 53, was admitted to the hospital for extreme weight loss, confusion, lethargy, inability to walk, and difficulty swallowing. On admission, she was somewhat confused, a vague historian and not forthcoming about her past medical history. Most of the history was obtained from prior outside hospitalization records and a sister.

The patient's medical problems seem to have commenced about 5 years prior to presentation. She reported that her weight was "normal" at about 150 pounds until that time. By her report, over the previous 5 years her weight steadily declined. She stated that 4 months previous to admission, her weight was about 120 pounds. At presentation she weighed 90 pounds.

A month prior to the hospitalization, the patient was admitted to another hospital for weight loss, gait instability, and confusion. Workup there included an unremarkable CT scan of the abdomen, pelvis, neck, and chest. She was noted to have transaminitis (elevation of transaminases i.e. alanine transaminase (ALT) and aspartate transaminase (AST), both important as indicators of liver disease) and a positive hepatitis C serology. She also had a TSH of 19 (normal 0.4–4 ml/L) and a free T4 level of 0.9 (normal 0.8–2.8 ng/dL). Total T3 was slightly decreased at 57 mg/dL (normal 87–157). She was started on low-dose levothyroxine at 25 mcg per day. The patient also underwent an upper endoscopy and colonoscopy. Both were normal. Her symptoms were attributed to malnutrition and hypothyroidism. Her confusion and gait improved during a brief hospitalization and she was discharged home.

After discharge the patient continued to have a poor appetite described by her as "no energy to eat" and trouble swallowing. She continued to lose weight, becoming increasingly emaciated. She had been unable to eat any food for 3 days prior to the admission. Her sister bought her groceries, but she would only eat soft foods including a small amount of salmon and some steamed vegetables. On the day of admission, the patient's sister found the patient confused and so weak that she was unable to get out of bed.

At admission the patient was considered malnourished and was started on a high-dose thiamine 500 mg/day IV, as well as folic acid and multivitamins. She was noted to be hypothermic and bradycardic. On evaluation she was found to have mild dysphagia. She was able to swallow liquids but had more difficulty with solids. Her food intake was estimated to be 25% of the food she was offered. The hospital staff reported that the patient intermittently refused medication and was often uncooperative with nursing care. Ms. Y said she continually felt satiated and constipated and reported that "even soft food was not going down." She said that "nothing was passing through" to her stomach, and her intestines felt "constricted." I was brought into the case serving as the neurological consultant.

Ms. Y reported that she was confused at times and had blurry vision (but no clear-cut diplopia), numbness in her legs, and difficulty in walking. She described generalized weakness. She (implausibly) denied feeling depressed, suicidal, or excessively anxious. There was also no history of headache or episodes of loss of consciousness. Ms. Y emphatically denied currently drinking alcohol in spite of a history of prior alcohol abuse. She denied any prior eating disorder or bulimic-type symptoms. She was very concerned about her appearance, continually saying, "look at me" (at times tearfully). On questioning she did not acknowledge believing that she was too thin.

As a younger woman, she was reportedly healthy. She attended college on an athletic scholarship. She was always considered underweight based on expected BMI. After college she had a short-lived marriage which ended in divorce. While reporting that there was no violence in her marriage, she repeatedly complained that her husband had been "very controlling." She did not have children. She generally worked in retail-type jobs.

10 years prior to admission, the patient's father died. Her sister reported that the patient "went to pieces" afterwards. Their mother was eventually placed in a board and care facility, and according to the sister, the patient also had a great deal of difficulty dealing with her mother's decline.

Although the patient denied problems with anxiety or depression, there is evidence to the contrary. According to the sister the patient had a long-standing history of alcohol abuse that included a DUI arrest. The patient (who was clearly not a reliable historian) insisted that she has not had any alcohol since her arrest.

The sister reported that the patient had "had issues regarding food for years" and had always been "very picky eater." For example, she started a gluten-free diet despite lack of evidence of celiac disease. The patient denied this history and explained that her poor food intake was due to difficulty swallowing. While there is some history to the contrary, she also denied any symptoms of bulimia nervosa including a history of dental erosions (from forced vomiting.) According to her sister Ms. Y exercised excessively. The patient, agreed that "this could be possible."

Past medical history was notable for hepatitis C, hypothyroidism, and chronic constipation. Her medications on admission included levothyroxine 25 mcg daily, polyethylene glycol, and docusate sodium.

She was cachectic. She was first encountered lying in bed. Physical examination showed blood pressure 124/98 mm Hg, SaO2 100% on room air, pulse 40–50 BPM, respirations 18/min, and temperature 36.1 F. HEENT showed severe temporal wasting and a large goiter. She was not forthcoming to questions, answering only reluctantly and with flat (impassive) affect.

Mental status examination revealed that the patient was oriented x3. Naming of objects was normal with aid of repetition and three-step commands. Speech was fluent. She was able to count backwards from 20–1 and was up to date on some current affairs. There was a slight intention tremor on the right side. She had a slight drift bilaterally in the lower extremities. Her extremities showed diffuse muscle atrophy but no fasciculations. The lower extremities had a stocking-glove distribution loss of light touch and painful stimuli. Position sense was also slightly diminished in the lower extremities. Deep tendon reflexes (DTRs) were 3+ throughout except at the ankles, where reflexes were absent.

MRI scan of the brain from previous admission showed diffuse atrophy, slightly out of proportion for age. There were focal areas of encephalomalacia seen on T2 signals in the high midline cerebellar regions as well as the right cortical frontal area. There was also evidence of FLAIR abnormalities in the bilateral corona radiata. Her putamen was slightly hyperintense bilaterally. The findings were nonspecific and could represent old head trauma, strokes or demyelinating, or inflammatory disease. Chest X-ray showed atelectasis.

Laboratory studies included calcium high at 70.6 U/mL (9–29 normal), HIV screen negative, TSH 15.3 mIU/L, total T3 of 2.97 mg/dL, free T4 slightly high at 1.58 ng/dL, sodium 136 mEq/l, K of 3.9 mEq/l, BUN 60 mg/dL, creatinine 0.65 mg/dL, magnesium 2 mg/dL, WBC count 7200 per mcL, hematocrit 35.2%, platelets 53 per mcL, ProBNP (brain natriuretic peptide, used to diagnose heart failure) 514 pg/mL [high], Utox negative, alcohol negative, ALT 240 IU/l, AST 156 IU/L, albumin 2.9, and total protein 6.1 g/dL.

The impression at this time was that the patient had the stigmata of severe malnutrition including cachexia, muscle wasting, signs of nutritional deficiency, skin dryness, bradycardia, transaminitis, and thrombocytopenia. Her neurologic findings of confusion, gait instability, generalized weakness with muscle wasting, and peripheral neuropathy could all be explained by her malnourished state and related vitamin deficiencies. In summary, the unifying basis of this patient's presentation was likely (unconfirmed) anorexia nervosa, with underlying major depression exacerbated by hypothyroidism. However, given that there was no prior diagnosis of an eating disorder, a more complete workup to exclude other causes of her neurological presentation and weight loss was needed. Possibilities included an occult malignancy (a CT scan of the chest, abdomen, and pelvis was already done and negative for malignancy), an associated autoimmune disorder such as Hashimoto's thyroiditis with encephalopathy, and ongoing alcoholism. An added possibility was neurodegenerative disease given the white matter findings on MRI and the areas of encephalomalacia, although the latter could have been related to undisclosed prior CNS trauma.

A B12 level, a cervical and a repeat brain MRI with and without contrast to look for any other areas of white matter disease and signs of inflammation, Hashimoto's thyroiditis laboratory studies, Cortrosyn stress test (to assess adrenal function), basic rheumatological panel, EEG, and a formal fasting study were ordered. Psychiatry, rheumatology, endocrinology, and oncology consults were ordered. The patient was maintained on thiamine, folate, and multivitamins. The hospitalist service started the patient on TPN (total parenteral nutrition). However, the patient refused ALL new studies, saying she was concerned about her appearance and did not "want to be seen" when taken to have the tests performed.

Ms. Y continued to eat only small amounts of food complaining, "I'm very constricted inside." Psychiatry evaluated the patient and confirmed the diagnosis of anorexia nervosa. A second swallow study demonstrated no abnormalities of swallowing and no obstructive pathology involving her esophagus. A celiac disease panel came back negative as did her lupus antibodies. Her thyroid peroxidase levels were high at 59 Iu/mL, and her NT TPO (antithyroid) antibodies returned positive. Based on these studies she was diagnosed with Hashimoto's thyroiditis by endocrinology. Hashimoto's encephalopathy could not be excluded without the repeat MRI with contrast and lumbar puncture, which the patient refused. As an urgent measure it was therefore decided to give the patient an empiric trial of IV corticosteroids to treat Hashimoto's encephalopathy.[1]

At this point the patient surprisingly agreed to an EEG (electroencephalogram) which demonstrated a slow background rhythm with intermittent right frontotemporal sharp waves. Given the history of intermittent confusion on presentation, the patient was started on empiric levetiracetam for seizure control.

In the hospital the patient was observed to have what appeared to be several generalized tonic-clonic type seizures. However, there was no postictal confusional state recorded, and there were reports of the patient being awake through the seizures. During one of these episodes, she was observed by neurology to have generalized body shaking but no eye movement abnormalities; she retained control of her arm when it was placed above her head and stopped shaking on command. It therefore was conjectured that the seizures were likely nonepileptic in origin.

Later in the admission, when finally receiving TPN, the patient was less confused but still continued to refuse diagnostic studies without coherent explanations other than being concerned about her appearance. With considerable daily persuasion, the patient eventually consented to a lumbar puncture and MRI of the head and neck with contrast. The lumbar puncture was essentially negative, and the MRI did not demonstrate any new enhancing lesions. The steroids for Hashimoto's thyroiditis were therefore stopped.

The patient continued to refuse any oral medications. She continued on TPN feeding taking very little by mouth and was generally observed pacing or fidgeting. At this point, 14 days after admission, with no improvement in her oral intake and no significant weight gain, the treatment team decided that nasogastric (NG) tube feeding would be appropriate. The patient, however, refused tube feedings. She continued to fixate on her weight and appearance and did not embrace the suggestion that her weight loss and preoccupation with weight might reflect anorexia nervosa. She was preoccupied with being unable to swallow and constipation. She was gen-

---

[1] Patients with Hashimoto's encephalopathy respond dramatically to steroid therapy. The initial dose of steroids varies between 50 mg and 150 mg of prednisone daily and usually slowly decreased over weeks to months, depending on the clinical course. While rapid improvement can be observed within 1–3 days, the average time from start of therapy to significant clinical improvement is 4–6 weeks. [1].

erally agitated and uncooperative. The psychiatry consultant who was following the patient felt that she had become delusional based on her bodily distortions and her inability to use sound judgment.

As the neurology consultant I felt that the patient was exhibiting diminished capacity to make medical decisions. Her sister was willing to act as a surrogate decision-maker, however. With the sister's consent, an NG tube was placed for the purpose of maintaining nutritional status. The hospitalist, however, canceled the order, holding that the patient could not be mandated to eat and had the right to refuse artificial nutrition. A different hospitalist who came on the next day was able to talk the patient into having an NG tube placed, and tube feedings were again initiated. The patient tolerated the NG tube for about 2 days but then pulled it out and refused replacement. The hospitalist service was unwilling to replace the feeding tube against the patient's will despite the finding of decreased decisional capacity.

By 3 weeks, despite TPN, the patient had lost 2 pounds from her admission weight and continued to have limited comprehension of her situation. Attempts to get her admitted to an inpatient eating disorders psychiatry program were unsuccessful due to insurance restrictions. Neurology and psychiatry continued to recommend that an NG tube be replaced and both services felt the patient was exhibiting diminished decisional capacity to refuse the treatment. The hospitalist service, however, continued to resist placing an artificial feeding device in this (decisionally impaired) patient who was refusing the treatment.

A bioethics consult was obtained. The bioethics committee met, and the hospitalist physicians were invited to participate. The committee was unanimous in concluding that the patient was exhibiting impaired capacity to make medical decisions. She was confused, delusional, did not fully comprehend her diagnosis, and could not fully understand the risks and benefits of the treatment she was refusing. The committee concluded that the patient's condition was essentially life threatening and that medical intervention did not require her to demonstrate intact decisional capacity.

In summary, this patient exhibited severe mental impairment and had diminished decisional capacity. Her medical status was potentially reversible with treatment. The committee suggested that the sister act as the surrogate for consent while court ordered conservatorship was obtained. The sister declined continued involvement at this point citing her frustration with the situation. The bioethics committee accepted responsibility for decisions about the patient's care and granted permission to start tube feeding. Conservatorship was eventually obtained. After the bioethics committee meeting, the hospitalists involved conceded that the bioethics process had been helpful and educational and provided the support they felt they needed for decisions made.

Follow-up: With tube feedings the patient's weight increased. Her confusion, weakness, and gait instability improved. With time she seemed to have more insight into her disease. Approximately 6 weeks later an inpatient anorexia nervosa program was found that accepted Ms. Y for transfer.

Reflections by Author

On reflection, this patient exhibited multiple levels of complexity. With no clear history of anorexia nervosa, other etiologies for her weight loss and cognitive impairment needed to be excluded. Broad testing in this sort of case commonly yields results of unclear significance. In this case, for example, there were antibodies associated with Hashimoto's thyroiditis but no other evidence of that disease. Complicating matters was the patient's impaired cognition. She was preoccupied with her appearance and had delusional thinking leading her to refuse workups needed to substantiate or rule out critical diagnoses.

Refusal of NG feedings and perceived difficulty swallowing placed Ms. Y in a medically precarious position. She was constantly agitated, constantly pacing and fidgeting, resulting in further weight loss and clinical decline. Complicating matters further, Ms. Y's medical insurance refused to pay for treatment at a psychiatric facility for treatment of eating disorders when this was first proposed. Her treating physicians were left with only two options: force-feed the patient or continue to watch her decline. (Note, that even TPN feeding is not a long-term option for nutrition and has associated risks, particularly infection.)

At the heart of this case, is the often difficult issue of discerning what constitutes decisional capacity in medical matters and under what circumstances decisional capacity becomes compromised. Associated with this challenge may be the need for clarity about a complex patient's medical and psychological contributions that complicate his or her own clinical situation. An additional contribution may be related to customary indications for undertaking critical medical procedures. In this case, forced feeding with an NG tube was considered unacceptable by some of the treating physicians and imperative by others. Those opposing believed that tube feeding was acceptable mainly for patients with clear alterations in consciousness or brain damage such occurs in strokes. This patient, however, was conscious and able to speak. She was rational at points but had fixed delusional ideas about weight loss and food intake.

In this case, disagreement developed between hospitalists and the rest of the clinical team, including the psychiatrist and neurologist. The hospitalists felt that because the patient was somewhat oriented and at points rational she had decisional capacity. The counterargument was that the patient lacked decisional capacity since her delusions were not allowing her to fully comprehend the treatment being offered and its associated risks and benefits. If the patient lacked capacity, what level of treatment could she refuse? She had refused MRIs, EEGs, lumbar punctures, and blood tests. Some refusals were ostensibly rational, for example, not wanting a lumbar puncture because of the risk of headache. On the other hand, refusing tube feedings and not eating despite the risk of death were dangerous to her survival. The hospital bioethics committee provided the required guidance, tube feeding was initiated, and court ordered conservatorship was obtained.

Complexity Summary

1. Biological (including genetic)
   Acute:
   - Over the previous 5 years, the patient's weight steadily declined. There was a precipitous change during the previous 4 months. She stated that 4 months previously, her weight was about 120 pounds. At presentation she weighed 90 pounds.
   Chronic:
   - Patient's condition deteriorated affecting the quality of her thinking as she became cognitively impaired (unable to think clearly) and delusional.
2. Psychiatric/psychological
   - The patient had anorexia nervosa and a delusional disorder. Delirium and dementia had been ruled out. The patient had a history of alcoholism that included (we believe) several DUIs. Her reporting was continually contaminated by distortion and denial of fact. It is hard to know how volitional this was, but it does fit with a background of addiction.
3. Social (including family and other support systems)
   - Patient was partially estranged from her sister. No other friends or relatives are mentioned as being significant in her background.
4. Care delivery, including access to care
   - Insurance provided support for her general medical care, not initially for treatment of her anorexia nervosa. Obtaining adequate medical support for treating her anorexia nervosa was a struggle.
5. Fundamental factors supporting or obstructing the treatment, in particular quality and continuity of the physician-patient relationship
   - The only significant supporting person in Ms.Y's life, her sister, became disillusioned with the unrelenting nature of her difficulties and eventually distanced herself from the treatment. Disagreement between the hospitalist staff and her consulting physicians made intervention by the hospital ethics committee necessary for a lifesaving intervention. The three major factors obstructing this treatment were (1) the patient herself as she refused necessary medical interventions and workups, (2) her sister when she backed away from the patient's care, and (3) the hospitalist staff's reluctance to follow the wishes of the consulting physicians and their apparent lack of understanding of what constitutes capacity for medical decision-making. With persistence on the part of the consultants and the intervention for the bioethics committee clarifying the legal and ethical issues of the case, the patient's treatment could be brought to a satisfactory completion.

Reference

1. Kothbauer-Margreiter I, Sturzenegger M, Komor J, et al. Encephalopathy associated with Hashimoto thyroiditis: diagnosis and treatment. J Neurol. 1996;243:585–93.

Chapter 19
Sleep Apnea Treatment Refusal, Grandiosity and Suicide

Mehrdad Razavi, Thomas W. Miller, and Wendi Eden

This 47-year-old patient's unrelenting denial of illness prevented his compliance with treatment in spite of active medical surveillance. With serious conditions such as those encountered in this case, namely psychosis, and chronic medical disorders such as obstructive sleep apnea and diabetes mellitus, continuity of care over time with the patient and physician working in alliance is key to desired outcomes. Treating providers in this case were limited to a sleep specialist and primary care provider/nurse practitioner. Referral to a psychiatrist proved impossible. Apparently this patient's attachment to the sleep specialist permitted him to continue office visits, although even this connection was tenuous at best and did not prevent ultimate suicide.

On the last day of his life, 47-year-old MW woke up with determination, his objectives unknown even to his wife, friends, and family. An accomplished man, MW was deeply troubled. He was being treated for depression and anxiety when he entered my practice. His medical conditions also included diabetes mellitus, hypertension, and hyperlipidemia. He had intermittently been on a complex regimen of medications including metformin, glyburide (2 mg PO BID), metoprolol (50 mg PO

M. Razavi, MD (✉)
Innovative Sleep Centers, San Rafael, CA, USA
e-mail: Drrazavi@innovativesleepcenters.com

T.W. Miller
LightHouse Family Clinic, Ocean Shore, WA, USA

Currently at Innovative Sleep Centers, Aberdeen, WA, USA
e-mail: WMiller@innovativesleepcenters.com

W. Eden, TPSGT, RST
Innovative Sleep Centers, Redding, CA, USA
e-mail: Weden@innovativesleepcenters.com

© Springer International Publishing AG, part of Springer Nature 2018
S.A. Frankel, J.A. Bourgeois (eds.), *Integrated Care for Complex Patients*,
https://doi.org/10.1007/978-3-319-61214-0_19

twice daily), atorvastatin (40 mg PO daily), paroxetine (20 mg PO daily), risperidone (0.5 mg PO daily), and lamotrigine (100 mg daily, which was discontinued due to a skin rash). He was also supposed to be using a CPAP machine at night to manage his sleep apnea. However over the previous few months, he inexplicably stopped using CPAP and stopped caring about his life in general. His marriage suffered and he lost his job. On that bright winter day, however, MW did have a purpose, and it was not to seek help. He simply drove to a hardware store, bought a gun, and ended his life.

I first met MW at the request of his wife. He was receiving medical care 40 miles from his home, but his wife was looking for a primary care physician closer to home. On presentation he stated that he did not trust doctors. I responded with humor stating that since he would receive treatment from myself and a nurse practitioner, he would be "safe." He relaxed.

His past medical history included hypertension, hyperlipidemia, depression, and panic disorder. At times his panic disorder was so severe that he required emergency room visits. Currently, he was being treated with metoprolol 50 mg daily, paroxetine 20 mg daily, risperidone 0.5 mg twice daily, and alprazolam 0.5 mg three times daily as needed. MW had a family history of coronary artery disease and myocardial infarction on both his father and mother's side, but no history of psychiatric illness.

MW was an overweight (BMI of 32 kg/m2) but fit looking middle-aged man with a rotund face, a short neck, and a small airway, all compatible with obstructive sleep apnea. I also noticed clubbing of his fingertips bilaterally. His laboratory studies from our office included a fasting glucose of 234 mg/dL and an HbA1c of 9.4%. His EKG was normal. I recommended some additional laboratory studies (CBC, CMP, cholesterol, TSH, and testosterone) which he declined.

As we talked, it became clear that he had led a very productive early life that included many hobbies including photography, golfing, and woodworking. A software engineer by trade, MW had psychiatrically fallen on hard times, however. When I met him he was feeling "hopeless," had trouble sleeping, snored endlessly, and woke frequently with headaches. He complained of "lowness" and "lack of focus." He had arrived at a point where he could not finish a single project. These states of mind had affected his marriage and work. He alluded to experiencing "some psychiatric issues" throughout his life. When I pressed this subject he, however, objected and almost walked out of the room. After a few moments he calmed down and we concluded our talk. He stated that he was here "for his wife" and "would probably not be around for long." When queried about that statement he stated that he had no intentions to commit suicide. Nonetheless, his statement was so alarming that I told him that I was concerned for him and would like to refer him to see a psychiatrist. He declined.

As soon as he completed the blood tests, I pressed him for a sleep study, cardiac stress test, and chest X-ray (I felt compelled to provide a basic level of primary care typical for specialists in the rural community in which I was practicing). Sadly, he declined these as well. We decided to continue his current medication and to add metformin (500 mg twice daily). I advised him that antidiabetic medications could potentially drop his blood sugar to dangerous levels. I had my assistant educate him on the proper use of his home glucometer scheduling him for twice a day capillary blood glucose checks to verify compliance and effectiveness.

At the end of our appointment, I again told him I was worried about him and asked him to come in for a follow-up in 2 weeks. He stated that he would think about it and started to leave. Since I had been unsuccessful in obtaining his commitment for my most urgent clinical goals including his cooperation with sleep study and follow-up, I decided to press these matters more forcefully. As I was leaving the room and he was putting his clothes on, I stopped and asked, "tongue in cheek, what do you have against sleep?" He said "I love sleep and would like to get more." After a short discussion and an angry outburst directed at him from his wife, he acquiesced and the referrals were made. A small victory, but potentially meaningful, nonetheless.

At my next visit with MW, his home blood glucose readings were improved to an average of 115 mg/dL. Shortly afterwards, he had his sleep study, which showed severe obstructive sleep apnea (OSA) with a breathing disturbance index, i.e., apnea/hypopnea index (AHI) of 51 (normal value is below 5). That is, he had significant problems breathing during sleep, interruptions occurring almost every minute, each time lasting for about 10 seconds, accompanied by an oxygen desaturation nadir of about 84% (normal value is above 95%). He had no record of REM sleep prior to treatment but subsequently showed REM during his CPAP titration. He was treated with CPAP at 9 cm, the necessary pressure to normalize his breathing at night. He was subsequently monitored and compliant with treatment at 1 month follow-up.

I did not see him back for several months. At the return visit he brought two pictures that he had framed and matted as a gift for me. The pictures showed the ocean and depicted serenity that he said he lacked. I noted that the clubbing of his fingers had started to correct itself. He said he wanted to express his "gratitude" for my referring him for CPAP. He stated that to that point he "had never been as focused" and was "feeling great." He said, the last time he felt "that great" was when he was 20 years old. He then stated, however, in a way that peaked my concern since it seemed grandiose, that he had started a project that would be "bigger than Google." He said he was involved with investors and was "exceedingly confident." He attempted to reassure me further by saying that now he was fully focused on his "goals."

MW did not show up for his follow-up lab tests or appointments for several months, when he finally agreed to come in for me to monitor his hypertension, diabetes mellitus, and sleep apnea. He insisted that he was working ceaselessly on his new project and that it was "extraordinary." He said he was still using the CPAP, but he had not followed up with the sleep lab. He added that he was starting to wean himself off all of his medications. I warned against this but he stated that he was "confident" that he would be "fine." I advised him to follow up with the sleep laboratory, continue with CPAP and his medications, and follow up with me in 3 months for laboratory work and review. There was little arguing with him.

His next visit on was arranged at the insistence of his wife. According to MW, he was still using his CPAP machine and his anxiety was under control. I asked if he had a follow-up with the sleep clinic. He said "no." He continued to refuse recommended laboratory tests. I asked about blood sugars at home. He said he had stopped monitoring these as his time was "too valuable," and his partners were pressuring him to complete work. I was alarmed about his cavalier attitude about his medical care. After drawing the blood samples myself, I asked him and his wife to return for a follow-up visit in a few days. They agreed.

A few days later on March 28, 2013, he and his wife came for review of medications and a discussion about recent mood and cognitive changes. His condition had sharply deteriorated, and it became clear that his thinking, including his claims about his business activities, was delusional. His grandiosity was striking and he had become paranoid about some business associates. From a sleep perspective, he was having nightmares and according to his wife was snoring and gasping for air during sleeping again. He admitted to being depressed but denied suicidal ideation. The review of his labs indicated his diabetes mellitus was starting to spiral out of control. His blood sugar was elevated to above 350 mg/dL, and his Hgb A1c was back above 11.0%. I confronted him with my impression that he was not using his medication or CPAP machine.

At the next visit, he complained about overwhelming anxiety, trouble focusing, and leg pain. His examination was unremarkable except that the clubbing had reoccurred. I was alarmed again and was running a list of psychiatrists through my head, but the closest was 75 miles away. Nonetheless, I insisted that he see a psychiatrist to evaluate his mood disorder. To my dismay, he became incensed and refused. Feeling quite unsettled I nonetheless increased his risperidone to 1 mg BID and scheduled a follow-up visit with the sleep lab. My plan, until he engaged psychiatric treatment, was to stay in close touch with the patient and his wife through regular follow-up appointments. However, he then disappeared, not responding to our communications over the next few months. We heard several stories from others in the community that he had left his wife, had become a recluse, and then had moved to a distant city.

At my last visit with MW, he complained of chest pain, denying shortness of breath and diaphoresis. He stated that he was having panic attacks. His EKG showed normal sinus rhythm. After this appointment he disappeared from our clinic.

Two months later, MW's wife came in for an "urgent" appointment for herself. She wanted me to make an immediate appointment with her husband since she was alarmed at the changes in his behavior. She reported that she had not heard from him for 4 days. She was frightened and promised to bring him in as soon as she could locate him.

However, again, this appointment never occurred. Days later, I found a note on my office desk instructing me to call the coroner. I did and was stunned to find that MW had taken his life. What I learned, after the fact, was that 6 days previously MW had driven very purposefully to a hardware store where he bought a gun, drove a short distance away, and shot himself.

Commentary by Author

It seems that the only peace that MW achieved during our care of him was the brief time he underwent treatment for sleep apnea. From the point of view of the specialists in our clinic who knew him, a negative turning point in MW's physical and emotional health could have been when he stopped using the CPAP machine. Untreated sleep apnea can lead to a series of cataclysmic events; e.g., lack of oxygen, increased catecholamines leading to increased blood pressure and heart rate, release of glucagon which would result in increased blood sugar, and finally sleep (including REM) deprivation resulting in worsening mood and even psychosis. These developments are associated with the body's fight or flight phenomena, foreshadowing potential disaster. Social difficulties and noncompliance with medications could logically accompany these changes. The public (and unfortunately most clinicians, still) are largely unaware of the importance of sleep for metabolism, mood, and overall health, which we hope to influence by writing this chapter.

It is difficult to determine whether CPAP noncompliance was the cause or the effect in this case. Did MW stop using CPAP, resulting in worsening mood and then noncompliance with medications, or was the patient a victim of his own grandiose wish for success; i.e., did he feel, as many patients do, "that CPAP is enough and I do not have to take my medications anymore"? Did he feel better with CPAP, resulting in premature discontinuation of his medications leading to psychiatric disruption, accompanied/followed later by CPAP noncompliance? Both are possible.

Further, did we fail to monitor compliance and get him the mental health resources in time? These are questions that can be debated both from a medical and an ethical perspective. We do not have an answer in this case but are reminded that we must be vigilant in the face of major changes in a patient's mental status.

At the time of writing this chapter, both clinicians and patients are able to monitor their own compliance in real time on their smart phone. Would MW be alive today, if this capability had been available when we began treating him? Maybe? Would he have been alive if we had a psychiatrist in town? Again, maybe. Or was the problem, neither lack of compliance monitoring, nor lack of access to mental health resources, but rather the issue of patient's will and acceptance?

It is impossible not to take some blame for MW's death. Why MW stopped complying with our assessments and treatments is a mystery that will always haunt us. His pictures still hang in the clinic. To ourselves they are a testament to brilliance never realized but always sought by him. In patient care, for each patient you lose, a piece of your soul goes with them. However, this kind of thinking is rarely productive. The solace is that those in the future who accept your help can potentially be saved through reference to patients you have lost.

Complexity Summary

1. Biological (including genetic)
   Acute:
   – Acute episodes of dyscontrol of chronic systemic illnesses
   Chronic:
   – Hypertension, hyperlipidemia, diabetes type II, obstructive sleep apnea

2. Psychiatric/psychological
   - MW presented with depression and anxiety, as well as racing thoughts and grandiose thinking, consistent with bipolar disorder and panic disorder. Bipolar disorder and panic disorder have high statistical risk of suicide, approaching that of major depression, irrespective of whether the patient has comorbid major depression. Suicide risk is higher in male patients and increases with age in middle and older age; the presence of significant systemic medical comorbidity increases suicide risk further. Hence, this patient could have been well served by ongoing psychiatric care in collaboration with his primary care provider and sleep specialist who were treating him for chronic systemic medical illnesses. Diabetes mellitus of significant duration, especially with neuropathic and vascular complications, has a significant risk of vascular dementia, which can be subtle on initial presentation.
   - He also presented with noncompliant behavior and intermittent denial of illness
3. Social (including family and other support systems)
   - Married with no children, he was stranged from his nuclear family. He had significant stresses in work performance which were likely exacerbated by his systemic and psychiatric illnesses.
4. Care delivery, including access to care
   - There was one clinic in his town, and in a nearby town (30 miles away) with several medical specialists and a few primary care providers. There was one hospital, and no psychiatrist within 75 miles. These logistical barriers to convenient care by specialists may have affected clinical outcomes.
5. Fundamental factors supporting or obstructing the treatment, including the quality and continuity of the physician-patient relationship
   - Please see Commentary at the end of the case narrative.
   - The patient's apparent denial of illness (or at least the severity of his illness) may have impacted his compliance with treatment and his successful coping with illness-related challenges. He was intermittently noncompliant for long periods of time in spite of active medical evaluations, including the described sleep study. With chronic conditions such as panic disorder, bipolar disorder, obstructive sleep apnea, and diabetes mellitus, continuity of care over time with the patient and physician working in alliance is key to optimized outcomes.
   - Note also that the treating providers in this case are the sleep specialist and a primary care provider/nurse practitioner. Apparently this patient's attachment to the sleep specialist permitted him to continue to present himself for office visits, although even this connection was tenuous at best. Referral to a psychiatrist proved impossible, and one can see the urgent rationale for effecting a strategy to facilitate primary care-based mental health care.
   - Counteracting the possibility of an ongoing relationship with treating physicians were this man's depression and bipolar psychosis. Physicians not trained in psychiatry can hardly be expected to deliver technically optimal psychiatric care in cases of this sort. The authors of this narrative deserve high praise for understanding that they served as a powerful barrier in delaying this man's suicide.

Chapter 20
Pain Management Progressing to Addiction in a Young Man with Quadriplegia

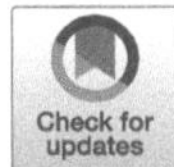

Deepak Sreedharan

Pain management became central to this case with the patient progressing from requiring oral opioids to IV opioids. His requirement for pain medication became unrelenting. The saga grew more complicated as his demands alienated not just hospital staff but his parents as well. The parents' marriage was tenuous with mother blaming the father for the patient's tragic competitive boating accident. Both ultimately blamed the hospital staff for their son's lack of progress. The author follows the patient's odyssey from legitimate pain management requirements to opioid addiction. The author discusses the management of pain through analgesic medication in some detail.

One of our local primary care physicians who has a solid reputation for managing all aspects of care by himself called me personally to refer Roger to my clinic. Seeing this doctor's name flash upon my cell phone meant I was being referred a challenging patient who would require significant time and energy, both of which are in short supply among physicians like myself. As one of the few pain management physicians in an area underserved by specialists, I am accustomed to being referred difficult cases. This case, where the assessment of pain was in question, challenged my attitudes about the routine use of opioids for management of reported severe pain. This case served as a reminder that even in the face of apparent suffering, the best course often is to exercise restraint with the use of opioids because of the risk that treatment itself can complicate the disease.

On the day of Roger's first appointment, I asked that he come just prior to lunch in anticipation of our spending more time than usual reviewing his case. When I went to meet him in the waiting room, I found a gaunt 21-year-old sitting patiently in a wheelchair with his father. Both were clearly uncomfortable. Although he was aware that I already knew a lot about his story, Roger went on to describe how he ended up in a wheelchair without any of the emotions or lack of detail I'm

D. Sreedharan, MD (✉)
Neurosciences, Sutter Health, 2800 L St, Sacramento, CA 95816, USA
e-mail: deepak.sreedharan@gmail.com

© Springer International Publishing AG, part of Springer Nature 2018
S.A. Frankel, J.A. Bourgeois (eds.), *Integrated Care for Complex Patients*,
https://doi.org/10.1007/978-3-319-61214-0_20

accustomed to hearing from patients with severe injuries and chronic pain. His seeming maturity and his ability to cope with his current state were remarkable.

He said that he was 17 years old and had no past medical problems. He had suffered a head and thoracic spine injury following a competitive boating accident. He had lost consciousness and required immediate intubation. At the hospital, he was diagnosed with a T5 spinal cord injury and underwent emergency decompression of his spine from T3 to T8 with fusion and instrumentation using pedicle screws. The force of the impact was enough to fracture his T5 and T6 vertebrae. Despite a valiant effort by his surgeon, postoperatively the patient remained a T5 paraplegic with residual pressure sensation but no light touch discrimination below T4. The patient was incontinent of urine and stool requiring periodic catheterization. He remained ventilator dependent and underwent bedside tracheostomy. Upon ventilator wean and reversal of his tracheostomy, the patient was transferred to a subacute rehabilitation center. It was during rehabilitation one and a half months post injury that the patient's chronic pain became manifest.

The patient was trialed on acetaminophen, muscle relaxants, and an SNRI (antidepressant/antianxiety drug). The SNRI was discontinued due to exacerbation of autonomic dysreflexia, precluding continued use of this class of pain medication. Since the patient had no prior history of recreational substance abuse, it seemed safe to next attempt escalating doses of opioids beginning with hydrocodone, then morphine, then a fentanyl patch before ultimately settling on IV hydromorphone for pain control. The goal of pain management was to facilitate rehabilitation. Once Roger had achieved independent transfer from his bed to his wheelchair and was deemed well versed in self-catheterization and hygiene, he was to be rapidly weaned off hydromorphone and sent home on acetaminophen, cyclobenzaprine, and morphine.

In my office 3 months post injury, he described sharp pain at the surgical site with paroxysms of shooting pain up and down his spine in addition to persistent low-back pain. There was no evidence of allodynia, hyperalgesia, or myofascial tension or trigger points in his low back. His pain was complicated by persistent T5 paraplegia, a neurogenic bladder with VRE colonization (Vancomycin-Resistant Enterococci), and autonomic dysreflexia.

Roger originally delivered the preceding history himself calmly, with apparent maturity, and without the emotion expected from a patient whose life had unraveled so abruptly. Perhaps the patient's apparent resilience was due to the solidarity of family's support at that time. His parents owned a successful international business, and his father, on first visit, seemed committed to obtaining any care needed to rehabilitate his son. I made a mental note to refer Roger to a psychologist for an evaluation since his injuries were so devastating. My first visit, otherwise, was focused on managing his pain.

Counterintuitively, 70 percent of paraplegics suffer from chronic pain despite extensive sensory loss. Most of this pain is due to mechanical back pain or nociceptive pain. Other sources of pain include neuropathic pain [40%] or visceral pain [40%] [2]. Nociceptive pain is often described as dull or aching in nature. Neuropathic pain is more burning or "electric" in nature and if due to the spinal cord injury occurs at or below the level of injury but never above. Neuropathic pain above the lesion if present is unrelated to the spinal cord lesion. Visceral pain can occur and often results from repeated bladder infections or bowel obstruction.

When managing chronic pain, there is a well-established schedule of analgesics that clinicians are advised to follow. First-line agents include non-opioid medications such as acetaminophen, non steroidal anti-inflammatory agents (NSAIDs), and muscle relaxants. If quality of life or function does not improve, short-acting opioids can be tried followed by a combination of long-acting or more potent narcotics. Upon each progression of the patient's regimen, there must be documented improvements in either quality of life or function.

Roger had already been escalated to potent opioids at the rehabilitation center. Since his analgesia was inadequate upon presentation, I opted to place him on acetaminophen, lidocaine patches, morphine, baclofen, and gabapentin. He was referred for in-home physical therapy, massage therapy, as well as for pain psychology consult. Lastly, he was re-referred back to his spine surgeon to assess the success of his spinal fusion 6 months postoperatively. I also wanted clearance from his surgeon before starting NSAIDs since some surgeons believe these inhibit bony fusion. I asked him to return in 2 weeks for a reassessment.

It would be 2 months before I would see Roger again. In the interim, his spine surgeon had deemed his surgery a success and following a repeat CT scan was confident his spinal fusion was solid, with no residual evidence of central or neuroforaminal stenosis nor hardware failure. His surgeon also delivered the unequivocal prognosis that Roger would remain wheelchair bound for the rest of his life. Though his care team and I had already conveyed this judgment to Roger, apparently he and particularly his father were seriously provoked by it. The two lashed out against their surgeon, expressed a lack of confidence in his competence, and chose to end ties with him.

What also came to light at this visit is that Roger had presented at the emergency department (ED) in order to obtain IV opioids to treat his allegedly intractable pain eight times in the previous 2 months. Neither the family nor the hospital reported these visits to me. Roger described intense pain at the surgical site that radiated both in cephalad and caudal directions. His pain was now complicated by the development of a decubitus ulcer. The claimed "overwhelming" nature of the pain reportedly caused him to "black out" for minutes to an hour at a time. During these blackouts the patient described his state as non-arousable, and claimed he would go into respiratory arrest. I witnessed one such episode in my office that day. Watching the episode unfold unexpectedly was stressful to say the least. We joked as little as a month later when I facetiously remarked that I had "come close" to giving him mouth to mouth resuscitation.

Working under the assumption the patient's episodes of unresponsiveness represented a vasovagal response (i.e., syncope involving a temporary loss of consciousness resulting from an acute fall in blood pressure) to severe pain, I felt my only option was to aim for greater pain control. This is a challenge commonly faced by clinicians with patients at risk for respiratory depression and who require the prescription of an opioid. In these situations, one chooses to act on the side of caution.

I performed an opioid rotation to hydromorphone at an equianalgesic dosage to his previously prescribed morphine. My intention was to slowly titrate the patient's dosage. I provided education to the patient and his parents on the proper use of the medication, the signs and symptoms of respiratory depression, and the administration of naloxone at home in the event of respiratory arrest. Meanwhile, I referred him to a neurologist to further assess the cause of his syncope. I sent Roger home from my office reluctantly with the plan I described above, hoping I had done the right thing.

One unexplained fact nagged at me, however. Why was Roger experiencing pain that lancinated cephalad (toward his head) from his surgical site? If this was neuropathic pain, his pain should be located at the level of his lesion or caudally (toward his feet), not cephalad. If it represented muscle spasm, why did he not demonstrate any evidence of myofascial tension on examination? In fact, he had no muscle tone from T5 downward, as one would expect.

One month later, I received the call that Roger had been readmitted to our local hospital for similar symptoms of intractable pain and syncope. The parents were at their wits end and insisted on an admission until a solution was found. Complicating this situation, Roger's parents were barely speaking to one another. Roger's mother intoned that prior to the accident, her son had been pushed by his father to continue to compete in speed boating despite her objections and several previous serious speed boating injuries. The father – recognizing the truth of his wife's allegations – bore tremendous guilt and was clinging to hope that his son would walk again. His son had the same fervent wish. The family was in disarray. The support system I pictured within the family did not exist. Further, in spite several referrals, neither parent had contacted the psychologist to whom they had been referred, presumably as a reflection of their minimizing the reality of their son's injury and hoping it might resolve by itself. Five months after their son's becoming paraplegic, his parents were unsuccessfully struggling to cope with their own personal tragedy, not to mention its serious financial consequences.

While in the hospital, an aggressive effort was made to identify the cause of Roger's syncope. A CT angiogram (computed tomography angiogram used to visualize blood vessels) ruled out a vascular cause, EEG ruled out seizures, and a Holter monitor ruled out both arrhythmia and a vasovagal response. We were baffled, unable to find a clear anatomic or physiological cause, leaving us to speculate that his syncopal episodes might be psychogenic. I have seen many patients with chronic pain experience pseudoseizures. With pseudoseizures, patients frequently manifest apparent convulsions as an emotional response to stress. The behavior is subconscious and involuntary. The usual signs, as was true in Roger's case, are a lack of EEG findings during episodes and lack of postictal confusion.

Additionally, Roger was likely demonstrating either addiction or pseudoaddiction. The distinction between addiction and pseudoaddiction is a subtle but important one. In addiction, a patient is deliberately seeking opioids for recreational purposes. In pseudoaddiction, the patient suffers pain and due to an inadequate response by the treating physician exaggerates his or her symptoms to gain greater access to analgesics. Effectively, the diagnosis hinges upon whether the patient's experience of pain warrants escalating the use of opioids. These situations are replete with uncertainty, in part based on contradictions between the patient's reports and medical assessment. After all, pain is a subjective experience. How can one be certain a patient with a spinal cord injury and decubitus ulcer is exaggerating their pain?

The assessment process begins by searching for objective evidence to explain the patient's symptoms. For Roger, on hospital readmission, a repeat CT scan was obtained demonstrating the same T5–T6 vertebral fractures with appropriate hardware placement, stable fusion, and no evidence of further pathology. An MRI was obtained of the patient's cervical spine as well and read as normal. A neurosurgical consult suggested the patient's pain likely stemmed from a poorly placed screw. To make the diagnosis would require performing a diagnostic injection whereby a local anesthetic agent is placed on the screw to see if the patient's pain temporarily disappears. Unfortunately, the procedure could not be performed until the patient's decubitus ulcer was healed because of the risk of translocating bacteria to the patient's spine. This unproven hypothesis at least provided a possible explanation for this patient's lancinating pain.

However, doubts increased based on observations of behavior that was inconsistent with the patient's reported pain. Nurses serve a valuable and reliable source of information in the hospital. By virtue of their role, they spend more time with a patient than anyone else and are in the best position to look for cues of addiction or pseudoaddiction. With Roger, the nurses reported hearing him regularly laughing on the phone or leisurely enjoying a ball game on TV when he believed no one was watching, only to claim "excruciating pain" when the staff was within earshot. In another instance, a nurse witnessed an episode of alleged syncope. She violently tried to arouse Roger but he did not respond. To expose his bluff, she "warned" Roger that if he did not awaken she would have to call a code blue which meant he could be intubated. Roger awoke immediately.

I looked for additional objective signs of pain. As a former anesthesiologist, I am trained to recognize pain experienced by patients while they are under general anesthesia. In response to pain, patients will experience elevations in heart rate, blood pressure, breathing rate, sweating, movement, or even evidence facial grimacing. These are involuntary responses to pain. They are so reliable that often if you provide enough analgesics to temporarily return these functions to normal the patient will wake up without pain. Roger seldom demonstrated these objective signs even while claiming he was in great pain. Other useful signs on examination of detecting feigned pain include pain with superficial palpation, lack of pain while the patient is distracted, and pain in a non-dermatomal location. These examination findings were largely positive in Roger's case. Further, in Roger's case I still could not explain why his pain traveled upward toward his head. If the cause of his pain had been an aberrant screw touching an exposed spinal nerve, it should have caused pain at or below the level of the screw.

Finally, I was also able to witness Roger's response to receiving IV hydromorphone, his preferred analgesic. Anesthesiologists are aware that IV hydromorphone takes 5–15 min to provide relief with very few exceptions. Roger would claim relief immediately, suggesting it was psychological effect he was experiencing.

From a psychosocial perspective, after 10 days of Roger's hospitalization, the family had reached the point of exasperation. They were unable or unwilling to personally care for Roger until his pain was under control. Roger was then transferred to a subacute rehabilitation facility for decubitus ulcer and pain management. Our hope was that once his ulcer healed, he could have the aberrant screw removed, and he would be a candidate for an intrathecal pump. An intrathecal pump allows the infusion of medications including opioids at micro-dosages directly to the spinal cord to treat pain. Doing so often reduces a patient's potential to develop side effects from these medications and counteracts the development of pseudoaddiction or addiction to them.

It was too early to proceed with an intrathecal pump, however. At this point the team had to make a judgment call. Was Roger's pain genuine, requiring dedicated pain management, or had he developed an addiction to narcotics, using them as a means of escape from coming to terms with his injury? This is typically a difficult decision to make and one that I have seen many clinicians avoid, especially those that are hospital based.

The general approach to pain management over the last two decades has been: if a patient describes pain that person is given progressively higher doses of opioids. Eventually, almost inevitably, in this scenario the patient will develop tolerance to the narcotic and require even greater doses. As a consequence, many young patients with devastating chronic injuries such as Roger's will after years experience a flare that requires exorbitantly high dosages of opioids leading to serious side effects such as intractable constipation, physical dependence, sedation, respiratory depression, and even death by overdose. With that said, there are some patients that do manage their pain well on high doses of opioids and for unclear reasons seldom require a dramatic escalation. These individuals in my experience represent a minority of patients.

After reviewing my findings with Roger's parents, we agreed to continue to provide Roger access to low-dosage oral opioids *only*, discontinuing IV opioids. By doing so we would be limiting treatment to only the baseline pain Roger was experiencing, setting limits that would prevent Roger from developing opioid tolerance and dependence. Eliminating his dependence on IV opioids also meant Roger was one step closer to returning home.

The confidence to reduce though not necessarily eliminate Roger's dependence on opioids is based on the opioid guidelines released by the Centers for Disease Control (CDC) in 2016 [3] encouraging the judicious use of opioids for chronic pain control. Unfortunately, the vast majority of patients will eventually develop tolerance to opioids. Over time, it is unlikely that the patient will experience any greater relief of pain on high doses than on lower doses of opioids. Also, by using higher doses of opioids, the patient will be placed at greater risk of complications. The most devastating of these are respiratory arrest and death. The CDC recently stated that the risk of serious overdose is two to three times greater at doses of 200 mg morphine compared to less than 60 mg of morphine. This risk increases to three to fourfold at doses greater than 300 mg morphine. Despite an altruistic desire to offer higher doses of an opioid to alleviate pain, treating physicians are reminded that at some point, the risks of treatment can outweigh the potential benefits. In these circumstances, as heart wrenching as it may be to wittness the patient suffering, it is better to explain to the patient that further escalation of opioids is not justified and focus must switch to alternative means for managing the patient's pain.

Fortunately, in the setting of spinal cord injuries, there are options. It may come as a surprise to many, but a growing body of evidence supports the value of conservative care options such as cognitive behavioral therapy, meditation, biofeedback, massage therapy, and hypnosis for pain relief and restoration of function [1, 2]. Often, these approaches can be more effective than opioid therapy used long term.

Hopefully, by setting limits on his access to opioids today and directing him to these alternatives, we will have set Roger on a better, more viable path. The greatest lesson I have learned as a pain management specialist involves acknowledging our current limitations in treating pain. Aiming for 100% pain relief is an unrealistic goal, and patients should be alerted to this fact early in treatment. As a summary statement, it is better to apply all the treatments we have in moderation, putting as much effort in limiting side effects as into achieving pain relief. Finding that balance with opioid therapy can truly save lives.

Complexity Summary

1. Biological (including genetic)
   Acute:
   - T5 spinal cord injury followed by emergency decompression of the spine from T3–T8 with fusion and instrumentation using pedicle screws. The force of the impact was enough to fracture the T5 and T6 vertebrae.
   Chronic:
   - Despite a valiant effort by his surgeons, postoperatively the patient remained a T5 paraplegic with residual pressure sensation but no light touch discrimination below T4. The patient was incontinent of urine and stool requiring periodic catheterization.
2. Psychiatric/psychological
   - The patient's limited tolerence of his handicap and the accompanying pain were not obvious at first. Initially the patient presented himself as "calm, with maturity, and without the emotion expected from a patient whose life had unraveled so abruptly." Over time his claims of pain became suspect as he required increasing doses of opioids. His calm demeanor was replaced by a style dominated by manipulation. Nociceptive (injury specific) pain was superseded by neuropathic (chronic) pain and claims of pain likely reflecting pseudoaddiction.
   - Comorbid depression is common in chronic pain states and could be screened for and monitored with standardized rating instruments. Noradrenergic-active antidepressants can be considered for adjunctive treatment of pain, even in the absence of a clear depressive disorder.

3. Social (including family and other support systems)
   - Significant family discord became apparent with the mother in particular blaming the father for the patient's accident. The family's tolerance for the patient's behavior wore thin, especially as his demands for pain control increased. The patient apparently also failed to comply with efforts at rehabilitation, with the development of decubitus ulcers a possible consequence.
4. Care delivery, including access to care
   - Care was transferred to a long-term acute care hospital as an effort to gain therapeutic control and as more conventional treatment progressively failed.
5. Fundamental factors supporting or obstructing the treatment, in particular quality and continuity of the physician-patient relationship
   - The patient's manipulations to obtain pain medication and his lack of compliance with treatment were discouraging to the medical staff who progressively became disaffected with a patient they originally championed. Family disillusionment and discord also played a significant role in hospital staff becoming disaffected with the patient. In addition, as the patient's failure to progress became intolerable to the parents, their blame toward his caregivers including his physicians grew.

While primary care physicians might be familiar with cases of this sort, understanding and managing the details of the relationship between the psychiatric, family, and systemic medical systems is challenging. In addition to a pain specialist, a treatment team that includes mental health professionals is required.

In summary, there were multiple sources of disunity in treatment in this case underscoring the need for the patient, family, and treatment team to work together in order to achieve a desirable outcome.

References

1. Cardinas D, Jensen M. Treatments for chronic pain in persons with spinal cord injuries. J Spinal Cord Med. 2006;29:109–17.
2. Cardinas D, Turner J, et al. Classification of chronic pain associated with spinal cord injuries. Arch Phys Med Rehabil. 2002;83:1708–14.
3. Centers for Disease Control (CDC). Guidelines for prescribing opioids for chronic pain. J Pain Palliat Care Pharmacother. 2016;30(2):138–40.

Chapter 21
Complex Regional Pain Syndrome (CRPS) and Progressive Medical and Psychiatric Deterioration

Alvin Lau

This is a highly detailed case of a young man with a progressive pain syndrome, following a discrete episode of trauma to his hand. The pain became increasingly complicated to manage, leading to many challenges to symptom control. As well, the attempted acquisition and coordination of highly specialized consultative services for a patient managed in a county health system was frought with difficulties. This patient's social isolation and low level of social function (significantly attributed to the chronicity of his pain) added to the challenges of delivering care focused on his pain syndrome and its many functional implications.

A 30-year-old man with complex regional pain syndrome (CRPS) and progressive medical and psychiatric deterioration is the focus of this case, illustrating the difficulty procuring medical resources and systemic problems within that health system.

Patients with chronic pain syndromes can be among the most difficult and challenging to manage given the relatively subjective nature of symptom severity, frequent psychiatric comorbidities, and concerns with chronic opiate therapy playing into or leading to an opioid use disorder. Many options for measuring pain are available. The most common include unidimensional pain scales such as the visual analogue scale, the verbal rating scale, or the numerical rating scale [1]. The wide number of available instruments along with lack of standardization for optimal performance of these instruments [2] leads to limited consensus about the most appropriate tool to use for clinically assessing pain. A strong multidisciplinary team is necessary for optimal care in these situations, but even then these cases can pose significant challenges, as illustrated by the following case.

Mr. T was a 30-year-old man with a 4-year history of complex regional pain syndrome (CRPS) who presented for evaluation in a county-operated primary care clinic. Complex regional pain syndrome (CRPS) is a chronic pain condition most

A. Lau, MD (⊠)
University of California School of Medicine, San Mateo, CA, USA

County Federally Qualified Health Center (FQHC), San Mateo, CA, USA
e-mail: alvinlau.md@gmail.com

© Springer International Publishing AG, part of Springer Nature 2018
S.A. Frankel, J.A. Bourgeois (eds.), *Integrated Care for Complex Patients*,
https://doi.org/10.1007/978-3-319-61214-0_21

often affecting one limb (arms, hands, legs, feet), typically occurring after an injury or trauma to that limb. There were initially two variants called CRPS-I and CRPS-II, with approximately the same symptoms and treatments. CRPS-I (previously called reflex sympathetic dystrophy) occurs in cases without identified nerve injury although causation is attributed to an initiating event (e.g., a crush, soft tissue injury, or immobilization), while the designation CRPS-II (previously referred to as causalgia) requires evidence of confirmed nerve injury. The International Association for the Study of Pain (IASP) criteria were initially proposed in 1994, and with subsequent revision in 2007 a third diagnostic subtype, "CRPS not otherwise specified" was recommended as well. Current diagnostic criteria (based on IASP proposed criteria) includes continuing pain that is disproportionate to any inciting event as well as multiple symptoms that may include sensory, vasomotor, sudomotor, motor, or trophic abnormalities or asymmetries.

Nonetheless, the pathophysiology of CRPS remains unclear. It is generally hypothesized that CRPS develops when persistent noxious stimulation leads to peripheral and central sensitization that lowers stimulus thresholds. Increased stimulus processing and response intensity leading to hyperalgesia and allodynia at the initial injury site can also expand beyond the initial region of pathology. Other hypotheses include sympathetically maintained pain, sensory and motor dysfunction, as well as abnormal healing and exaggerated inflammation which leads to increased protective disuse, promoting fear avoidance and potentially leading to a neurological neglect state. This syndrome most commonly affects people ages 20–35, involving women more often in men.

Research on CRPS treatment is ongoing, and new guidelines are continually being generated for diagnosis and treatment [3]. However, the uncertainty and complexity of the pathophysiology and diagnosis as well as low prevalence (20.57 per 100,000) [4] make CRPS a challenge to diagnose and treat in an evidence-based manner. Mechanistically, CRPS is conceived of as neuropathic in nature, so agents such as tricyclic antidepressants (e.g., amitriptyline), GABAergic agents (e.g., gabapentin, pregabalin), and/or other antiepileptics all qualify as options in treatment. Gabapentin is likely effective via enhancement of natural GABA systems in pain modulation but also possibly via suppression of excitatory amino acids such as glutamate. Other antiepileptic drugs may act via their membrane stabilization properties and thus may be especially indicated in scenarios where nerve damage or ectopic neural activity is involved in generating pain.

Apart from these medications, there are interventional therapies available for CRPS. Generally these include stellate ganglion blocks/lumbar sympathetic blocks, intravenous regional anesthesia, intravenous infusions, brachial plexus/spinal infusions, ablative sympathectomy (radio frequency/alcohol-phenol), and spinal cord stimulation. A local port for bupivacaine infusions can be used as a version of intravenous regional anesthesia. Unfortunately, studies indicate lack of efficacy of such treatments. Also, port implantation is unusual given the risks associated with an implantable foreign body for an unclear duration.

CRPS symptoms vary in severity and duration. Studies of its incidence and prevalence show that while most cases are mild and patients recover gradually with time. In more severe cases such as Mr. T.'s, patients may not recover and may have long-term functional disability. A county primary clinic or a regional mental health clinic such as the one where Mr. T., the patient described in this report, was being treated is unlikely to provide the sophisticated treatment required in these situations.

Mr. T's psychiatric history prior to surgery was negative by his report. His social history was notable for his having lived in Chicago before relocating to California. While there he studied for a law degree which he did not finish. Post-injury and during the initial development of CRPS, he moved to the San Francisco Bay Area ostensibly to complete law school and to be near his family. Unfortunately, conflict developed between the patient and family members. When the patient first encountered me, he had minimal family support and few friends. He had dropped out of law school leaving him with student loans that he was having difficulty paying off.

Mr. T. suffered a right hand laceration while living in Chicago 2 years previous to his presentation at our clinic. The injury was deep enough to sever the ulnar nerve and required surgical reattachment for repair. The circumstances of that injury were unclear. The patient reported that it was a kitchen accident associated with his having "fumbled unsuccessfully with a knife." Some of his mental health clinicians wonder if the patient's history may be inaccurate, indicating a possible self-injury component.

Mr. T. developed significant pain following surgery. He underwent multiple opioid treatment trials which were inadequate for controlling his pain. Eventually he received the diagnosis "complex regional pain syndrome" (CRPS). He reported receiving multiple medication trials and other treatments including stellate ganglion blocks. He eventually found a hand surgeon who placed two subcutaneous port devices so that he could self-inject bupivacaine near his ulnar nerve to provide pain relief. While this atypical treatment provided some temporary relief, associated complications had already arisen requiring the ports to be replaced. When the patient transferred to my care, his pain was controlled with bupivacaine injections as well as methadone 30 mg PO TID.

Since Mr. T.'s pain was controlled with the bupivacaine injections, I opted to see if we could discontinue methadone he was using to assist pain relief, believing that his bupivacaine was doing a more than adequate job of controlling his pain. Titration off methadone occurred without incident. He was switched to long-acting morphine sulfate. However, as the treatment continued over months the patient became depressed. In response, he was stabilized on an antidepressant regimen of citalopram 20 mg/day.

Over time, however, difficulties developed and the bupivacaine injections no longer controlled his pain. He returned to see a hand surgeon who did a direct ulnar nerve injection but with limited success. Fluoroscopy of the ports revealed that they were essentially shattered and occluded, rendering them useless. The patient now had two foreign bodies in his arm that provided no clinical benefit. With no medical relief available, his pain progressively worsened.

As Mr. T.'s primary care physician I initiated an additional series of medications in an attempt to stabilize his pain. The county primary care clinic was inadequately equipped to provide the broad range of services necessary for management of this patient's CPRS. Referrals were made to tertiary care centers for consultation and other assistance, but the patient was repeatedly rejected as ineligible for their services.

The patient's personal and social situation had become tenuous. At this point, the patient was homeless and living in shelters. He was unable to attend school because of his disability and had lost all money from his student loans. With pain worsening, his ability to cope with the day-to-day struggles from a chronic medical condition and difficult psychosocial circumstances had worn thin. When the port-injection treatments no longer provided relief, his pain, stress, and anxiety became manifest as sleep disturbance, fatigue, affective instability, and frustration. His relationships with other clinicians eroded. His lability, in the form of tearful frustration that at times turned into angry outbursts, was often directed toward clinic staff. He eventually transferred to a different regional clinic with the objective of achieving eligibility for county-sponsored housing nearer to the most desirable tertiary care center.

At this point, multiple additional treatment options were attempted. Even though the patient's pain was classified as "chronic non-malignant pain" (chronic non-malignant pain is defined as pain lasting 3 months or more or as pain persisting beyond the time of expected healing), opiates remained a mainstay of treatment. There was a possible muscle spasm component to patient's pain, so a muscle relaxant (cyclobenzaprine) was added. Given the vasospasm that temperature dysregulation can create under these conditions, I added calcium-channel blockers and beta-blockers but with limited success. Subsequently, we cycled through multiple combinations of new agents in an attempt to arrive at the best option. Switching of opiates was complicated given the variable efficacy and risk-benefit balance associated with each. I tried in general to adhere to a total daily opioid dose equivalent to 120 mg of morphine, since it appears that the analgesia-side effect ratios are less beneficial past that threshold. As one additional challenge, converting to and from methadone is difficult. Its nonlinear kinetics can make titration and conversion problematic. The short analgesia peaks versus long overall half-life of methadone make dosing difficult. Cardiac monitoring often becomes a necessity, especially when using it in concert with tricyclic antidepressants for neuropathic pain because of their effects on cardiac conduction. Further, fentanyl patches are more difficult to use than may be expected. Practical issues such as patch not sticking to skin and loosening of the patch during showering can make the patch, while an effective pain control option, impractical.

The primary care clinic in this situation was embedded (i.e., co-located) within a regional mental health center. In an effort to address the systemic medical comorbidity of patients with significant mental illness (SMI), embedding primary care services in a psychiatric clinic in effect attempts to "invert" the usual medical home model, with the mental health center serving as the primary location for health services. There are presumed advantages with this care model:

- Reduced stigma for patients
- Improved medical appointment adherence, including appropriate primary care screening

- Improved collaboration between psychiatry and primary care, including more "warm hand-offs," more immediate on-site evaluation of systemic medical concerns, and development a uniform psychiatric formulation
- Easier access to clinical information

Unfortunately, there are often unforeseen disadvantages to this particular care model as well:

- Embedding primary care service in a facility not specifically designed for those services translates to a less effective administrative support infrastructure, less appropriate clinical space, and less nursing support.
- Co-location to a clinic without a unified electronic health record for systemic medical and psychiatric care severely impairs information flow despite the ability to have a warmer hand-off between clinicians.
- Differences between the general medical and psychiatric formulary, insurance, and how prescriptions are handled in general can lead to confusion.
- Being farther removed from larger county medical clinics limits the range of on-site services available.
- Referrals still have to be sent to outside clinics.
- In part, as a consequence of these incongruities between primary care and mental health clinic protocols, questions were raised separately by the medical and psychiatric staff about the legitimacy of Mr. T.'s diagnosis. Staff members began to question whether his symptoms were in fact real, and there was a growing opinion that Mr. T. was being manipulative in repeatedly seeking medication for pain, suggesting an underlying comorbid personality disorder.

The imprecision about a diagnosis such as CRPS as well as lack of clinical experience can lead to clinicians' discounting symptoms and failing to appreciate a patient's distress. There were multiple times during the course of this patient's treatment when I was queried about the "legitimacy" of this patient's symptoms. Mr. T. contributed to staff concerns with his worsening depression, increased irritability/affective lability, and hostile dismissiveness toward staff members. All those factors contributed to his complex interaction with his mental healthcare team, breeding increasing distrust, splitting (his pitting one group against the other), and generally negative and distrustful attitude.

I was faced with the challenge of determining what I, as his primary care physician, should do in this highly challenging situation. Often primary care clinicians will defer to the opinions of their psychiatry colleagues about the psychiatric illness(es). But in this case, that option proved inadequate since the patient had alienated many staff members from both sides. In response, I contemplated whether I should have encouraged the patient and his mental health clinicians to meet together to review their interactions and come to a better understanding of each other's perspective. The alternative was for me to act as a release valve for the frustrations of both sides. I needed to avoid falling into a "split" dynamic among clinicians, whereby I could have either become overly dismissive of patient's symptoms myself or aligned with and overly encouraging of one faction.

Some of my strategies in this situation included:

- I built my own rapport with the patient, continually validating his frustration and concern.
- I validated my mental health colleagues' concerns as well. I reviewed the contradictory evidence about the patient's medical condition while taking the position that all of the clinicians' observations likely had merit.
- I served as an advocate for the patient by speaking with shelter management about extending bed stays, obtaining housing, and referring the patient out to tertiary care clinicians.
- I provided frequent appointment check-ins on the principle that these interactions would likely be experienced as supportive and help contain his catastrophic concerns. As mentioned earlier, there were myriad difficulties getting appropriate tertiary care services throughout the patient's illness course.
- There were complex pain management issues in part because the county pain management clinic had significant limitations. While it was an excellent multidisciplinary clinic equipped to do general medication management and staffed with psychologists and other psychotherapists, they were not comfortable working with the patient's CPRS diagnosis and could only offer medication management and not more invasive interventions.
- The hand surgeon who originally placed the ports eventually stopped returning calls, leaving me to sort out how to deal with the now non-functional implanted ports. In a non-enclosed system, especially when clinical services involve a patchwork between primary care physicians and specialists, specialists who feel they have exhausted their treatment options can choose to discontinue a treatment relationship leaving the primary care physician without support. Primary care physicians have limited options when such an event occurs.
- Referral to tertiary care in this case was fraught with roadblocks. Initial referral to the county's preferred tertiary care center's pain management clinic resulted in a minimally helpful consultation. Their consultant agreed that the CRPS diagnosis was possible, but they did not provide any further services or advice. Further, they made no concrete recommendations for optimizing the patient's medication regimen. Instead, the tertiary care center indicated they would be better able to treat the patient when his social situation was more stable and that any other interventional modalities would not be considered until then. They also recommended that the patient be assessed by a pain psychologist. However, while the patient was connected with the regional mental health center, the associated psychiatrist and psychologists were not versed in pain psychology and its management. There was a pain psychologist at the county pain clinic. However, the patient was not entitled to the services of that psychologist as he was deemed an inappropriate candidate for county pain management program given the complexity of his case.

See the following "commentary" for further discussion of this case.

Commentary by Author

This description illustrates the fractured nature of a public mental health service even within a medical setting. Not discussed, but clearly relevant, is how different funding sources for mental health and medical services determine which type of financial support can be made available to patients. Attempts to refer Mr. T. to a desirable tertiary care center was a 4-month process and required multiple reviews from insurance and medical officials. When the sought after second opinion took place after many months, however, the tertiary center was (ironically) unable to accept Mr. T for ongoing treatment because of lack of insurance approval beyond the single consultation.

As I hope you can see, care coordination is a complex and often challenging undertaking. However, this situation also holds even for relatively familiar, essentially noncomplex, chronic disease entities such as non-insulin-dependent diabetes mellitus.

In reviewing this case, it is startling to see the magnitude and variety of difficulties encountered. The patient's lack of a social support system played a significant role. The absence of significant collateral and family involvement in coping with a difficult disease exacerbated the patient's challenges. This deficiency was linked to myriad other difficulties including lack of additional financial support, problems navigating the multiple disparate care services (the availability of a care coordinator might have helped), fragmentation of information and instructions between these care services, lack of a unified longitudinal perspective and plan about the patient's care, difficulty with self-advocacy, and lack of an active coping supports to help alleviate psychological burdens that result from chronic disease.

Also, interfacing between different care systems was problematic. Lack of a uniform electronic health record between municipalities, between healthcare systems, and between specialty sites (despite working within the same system) led to remarkable inefficiency, including the inability to manage clinical data. So many opinions and choices made by clinicians who encounter these kinds of difficulties diverge because of these incomplete data streams.

As the primary care physician, I intermittently served as patient navigator, but with limited time and broader other responsibilities, I was unable to do so on a regular basis. However, perhaps that is analogous to a role physicians potentially serve in similar clinical situations: as master plan-makers, allocating responsibility for executing these plans to others on the healthcare team. This model for physician responsibility should be considered for future management of complex patients and complex cases.

Complexity Summary

1. Biological (including genetic)
   Acute:
   – The patient experienced acute and chronic pain in response to both noxious and non-noxious stimuli.
   Chronic:
   – The patient experienced chronic pain and associated functional limitations.
2. Psychiatric/psychological
   – Given the chronic nature of the patient's pain, he was in continual distress. The patient also had comorbid depression and anxiety, not uncommon in patients suffering from a chronic pain syndrome [5, 6]. These states of mind are sequenced in reciprocal cycles of pain, depression, more pain, and more depression. This sequence itself also often lends to development of pathological fear and avoidance. In turn, this situation may have exacerbated an underlying personality disorder (in this case a shift to being manipulative) impacting his care experience in a negative fashion and reenforcing his anxiety and depression.
3. Social (including family and other support systems)
   – Concrete social disadvantages, not uncommon in a Federally Qualified Health Center (FQHC) population, were prominent features in this case. Unemployment and lack of financial resources led to unstable housing and social dysfunction. Added were lack of robust health insurance and difficulties in access to care. The lack of significant social support and family involvement in coping with and managing a difficult disease accentuated the patient's challenges. Improved social support might have (1) helped the patient navigate disparate care services and (2) unify fragmented information and instructions. (3) It might also have assisted in providing a longitudinal perspective for the patient's care and (4) improving patient advocacy; overall providing active coping supports to help alleviate psychological burdens resulting from chronic disease. Healthcare navigators or similar guides might have been useful as surrogates for some of the responsibilities that require social supports.
4. Care delivery, including access to care
   – Enrollment in a county care delivery system while generally acceptable for more common primary care complaints is much less effective with complex diagnoses. Despite the presence in this case of parallel county systems of care for systemic medical and psychiatric illness, the two units did not communicate well or efficiently. Electronic health records were used, but with multiple EMR systems in play, a unified data stream for all providers was not available. When the patient needed advanced (tertiary) care for his pain syndrome, access to ongoing specialty care was delayed and was limited to a single consultation. As the primary care physician in this case, I was forced to find and attempt to provide adequate care in spite of limited time and resources.

5. Fundamental factors supporting or obstructing the treatment, in particular quality and continuity of the physician-patient relationship
   - Author's continued commentary: The patient was successfully attending law school before his condition became severe. His cognitive functioning seemed at least adequate throughout my involvement with him, and my observation was that he was initially able to communicate with me and other care givers in a reasonable fashion. I had the ability to schedule patient visits at a relatively high frequency, allowing me to address his physical and psychiatric concerns rapidly and early in his treatment. Given my engagement with the patient's mental health providers, I was able to educate them about the patient's underlying medical issues and advocate for him despite their difficult interpersonal interactions with the patient.
   - Fundamental to the maintenance of this treatment was my commitment to the patient and his care. I frequently had to advocate for the patient so that he would receive appropriate care and so that care would not be disrupted as clinical and administrative problems arose. Of equal or greater importance is the personal significance of the patient knowing that I was dedicated to his care. I believe this was a powerful, and perhaps the most powerful, factor in sustaining the patient's commitment to our treatment.

References

1. Williamson A, Hoggart B. Pain: a review of three commonly used pain rating scales. J Clin Nurs. 2005;14:798–804.
2. Hjermstad MJ, Fayers PM, Haugen DF, et al. Studies comparing Numerical Rating Scales, Verbal Rating Scales and Visual Analogue Scales for assessment of pain intensity in adults: a systematic literature review. J Pain Symptom Manag. 2011;41:1073–93.
3. Harden RN, Oaklander AL, Burton AW, et al. Complex regional pain syndrome: practical diagnostic and treatment guidelines, 4th edition. Pain Med. 2013;14:180–229.
4. Sandroni P, Benrud-Larson LM, McClelland RL, Low PA. Complex regional pain syndrome type I: incidence and prevalence in Olmsted county, a population-based study. Pain. 2003;103:199–207.
5. Cheour M, Ellouze F, Zine I, Haddad M. Beck inventory depression assessment in chronic pain patients. Tunis Med. 2008;86:1074–8.
6. Poole H, White S, Blacke C, Murphy P, Bramwell R. Depression in chronic pain patients: prevalence and measurement. Pain Pract. 2009;9:173–80.

Chapter 22
End-of-Life Management Where There Is Family Opposition to Physician Recommendations

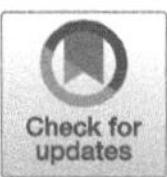

Curtis (Kip) Roebken

This patient at baseline was marginally functioning in his home. He underwent 4 months of hospitalization including 1 month in an ICU. During his multiple hospitalizations, he underwent tracheostomy and feeding tube implantations. He was unable to articulate his needs, other than to state that he wanted his physicians to "pull the plug." After he lost a friend to ovarian cancer, he was left with no personal support. His treatment course at this point was disrupted by the problematic involvement of his grandson who insisted on a home death and hired an attorney who was equally uncompromising. A struggle resulted that was ultimately resolved by the hospital comfort care committee and illustrates the medical and legal issues that these situations can pose.

Mr. T. was a 75-year-old gentleman who originally presented to our local long-term acute care (LTAC) hospital for an infected abdominal aortic aneurysm discovered during endovascular repair (graft) for that aneurysm. His background health and status was one of marginal independence. He was watched over by a neighbor who also happened to be an emergency medical technical and his grandson who lived in Chicago and communicated frequently with him but did not have a local presence.

A long-term acute care facility (LTACH) is a specialty care hospital designed for patients with serious medical problems that require intensive, complex treatment for an extended period of time (usually 20–30 days). Long-term acute care facilities offer more individualized and resource diverse care than skilled nursing, rehabilitation, or subacute facilities. Patients are typically transferred to an LTACH from intensive care units in short-term care facilities (STACHs). Short-term acute care hospitals are the hospitals whose services encompass the broad needs of critical patient care. Their services typically include emergency rooms, operating rooms, and full-service diagnostic facilities including imaging services (MRIs and CTs).

C. (Kip) Roebken, MD (✉)
Kentfield Long Term Acute Care Hospital, Kentfield, CA, USA
e-mail: kentdoc45@yahoo.com

© Springer International Publishing AG, part of Springer Nature 2018
S.A. Frankel, J.A. Bourgeois (eds.), *Integrated Care for Complex Patients*,
https://doi.org/10.1007/978-3-319-61214-0_22

An LTACH is an extension of this care, devoted to providing a continuum of services. CMS (Center for Medicare Services) has mandated that LTACH criteria for admission include a 3-day stay in an ICU or the need for continuing ventilator support.

To some degree, these designations represent a monetarily motivated response to the cost of support in the intensive care unit (ICU) environment. LTACHs can very effectively manage these patients as a part of a care continuum. The care continuum includes not only acute care hospitals but also skilled nursing facilities, subacute units, rehab facilities, home care agencies, community hospice, and of course family members able to participate in care when the home situation can be negotiated. Structurally the continuum must address the serious questions raised by escalating costs of care particularly for patients in the "boomer," aging population.

Mr. T.'s medical condition took a turn for the worse when he had a mechanical fall in his home. He lacerated his arm and shortly afterward was hospitalized for a methicillin-sensitive *Staphylococcus aureus* (MSSA) bacteremia. He was later discharged to a skilled nursing facility (SNF). A skilled nursing facility is a type of treatment facility organized by Medicare and Medicaid as meeting long-term healthcare needs for individuals who have the potential to function independently after a limited period of care.

While at the SNF, Mr. T. developed atrial fibrillation and abdominal pain requiring his referral to a short-term acute care hospital (STACH). On that admission, in 2013, he continued to complain of abdominal pain and had impaired cognition resulting from underlying infection and sepsis. He was found to have slippage of his endovascular graft and was taken to the operating room. Initially there was no evidence of aneurysm rupture and he was treated for atrial fibrillation. However, further follow-up imaging done because abdominal pain failed to resolve showed an increased size of his aortic aneurysm. He was taken back to the operating room and was found to have a ruptured aortic aneurysm with evidence of an infected endograft and purulence at that site, along with an aortoenteric fistula.

At this point Mr. T. required further extensive surgery that included removal of the graft. He was then transferred to the intensive care unit. Blood cultures again grew out methicillin-sensitive staph. He was not able to have a primary surgical closure of his wound because of its dimensions. He could not be weaned from assisted ventilation, and roughly a month after his presentation to this facility, he underwent a tracheostomy. During this hospitalization he also required right arterial-femoral bypass. He subsequently developed a hospital-acquired *Clostridium difficile* enteritis infection.

Mr. T. was a retired divorcee and had minimal personal support. He, as mentioned, had close ties to a neighbor who was an EMT (emergency medical technician). However, unfortunately, during his hospital stay, she was diagnosed with ovarian cancer and was unable to provide support for him or input for decision-making.

At this pivotal point, the patient was transferred to our LTAC for extended care. My involvement was that of an attending physician. Examination on admission revealed a gentleman who appeared very frail. His level of consciousness was stuporous. He would only occasionally nod his head to respond to questions. He could not follow commands except to open his mouth when that gesture was demonstrated to him by his observer. His vital signs were all reasonable with a temperature of 98.4 °F, an elevated heart rate of 112 BPM, a respiratory rate of 18/min, and a blood pressure of 104/78 mm Hg. Prominent physical findings included coarse rhonchi throughout his lungs (tracheostomy was in place). Irregular cardiac rhythm was noted with a systolic murmur. At that point he had a large ventral abdominal wound with sutures and a wound VAC in place. Prominent on his examination were ischemic necrotic digits involving all ten toes. He was found to be ventilator dependent with the prospect that he would require mechanical ventilation for the duration of life (consistent with our neurodiagnostic panel).

At this point we clearly were dealing with a highly complex patient. His issues included ventilator dependence, cardiovascular issues including congestive heart failure, peripheral vascular disease partially associated with his aortic abdominal aneurysm, infection stemming from a staphylococcal infection with hospital-acquired *C. difficile* enteritis, and necrotic toes. All LTACH resources were leveled at his care. He had the benefit on an infectious disease consultant as well as the ancillary services of physical therapy, occupational therapy, and speech therapy. Nursing and wound care were effectively delivered.

His progress was as follows. With diligent wound care, there was improvement of the abdominal wound. His mental status improved somewhat so he was able to mouth some words. Over weeks, he became inconsistently oriented to self (person), hospital (place), and date (time). However, his course was one of medical challenges. The fact that active support from family members was minimal added to the difficulty managing him medically and establishing care goals. He developed periods of congestive heart failure that required diuretic therapy, and he had an elevated B-type natriuretic peptide in the 5000 pg/ml range associated with congestive heart failure. He became hypernatremic with sodium as high as 151 mEq/L, largely due to diuretic intervention for his congestive failure state. Renal function surprisingly remained stable with a BUN of 33 mg/dL and a creatinine of 0.6 mg/dL. He remained chronically anemic with a hemoglobin of 8 gm/dL and a hematocrit of 25% range. Chest films intermittently showed pleural effusions associated with his congestive heart failure.

His treatment course at this point was epitomized by the final, disruptive events in his hospitalization and the problematic involvement of his grandson. During these last weeks of hospitalization, Mr. T. repeatedly requested that life support be removed. By that time, he was communicating quite clearly and accurately. He even mouthed the words "pull the plug."

Discussions were held with his grandson by phone. He was his designated power of attorney and became firm in insisting the patient be allowed to die at home. He was unable, because of distance and personal obligations, to be at Mr. T.'s bedside. Instead, the grandson hired an attorney to facilitate the interpretation of the patient's wishes, both grandson and attorney insisting that a home death be made possible. To this end, an independent palliative care physician in the area in which the patient lived was consulted by them as an advocate for their point of view. However, this consultant eventually declined to provide care when the defined goal of returning home and being taken off life support was made clear.

From an operational standpoint, it was felt by his attending physicians, including myself, that the patient did not have the physical capacity to allow for transfer to his home nor could his medications be adequately administered at home so that he could comfortably expire. Many of these people were sympathetic to the notion that the patient should be able to die at home but recognized that the proper supports were not available to allow this to happen safely. The attorney representing the patient and his grandson, however, grew adamant and insisted that hospice care made available in the patient's home. It is worth noting that conflicting goals between patient and family concerning home death frequently arise and complicate patient's end-of-life care.

Ultimately, this patient's case was brought before the comfort care committee at our hospital. All parties ideally wanted to carry out the patient's directive about cessation of life support. Unfortunately the ability to have this done in the home setting could not be accomplished either logistically or medically. Consequently, after much debate between the patient's attending physicians, his grandson and his attorney, this patient was taken off assisted ventilation and under morphine sedation quietly expired in the hospital setting.

Commentary by Author

This patient at baseline was marginally functioning in his home. He underwent 4 months of hospitalization, including two admissions to short-term care including 1 month in an intensive care unit (ICU). He spent 2 months at a skilled nursing facility (SNF) level of care before coming to us. Procedurally he had two major surgeries with resultant surgical wounds that needed to heal. He developed a hospital-acquired infection of *C. difficile* enteritis. A recurrent staphylococcal infection that originated in his home ultimately took his life. During his multiple hospitalizations, he underwent a tracheostomy and feeding tube implantation with the intention of improving his capacity to survive. While he originally was supported by a friend, she was forced to drop out of the picture after developing ovarian cancer. His treatment course at this point was epitomized by the final, disruptive events in his hospitalization including the problematic involvement of his grandson. His grandson insisted on a home death and hired an attorney who was equally uncompromising. A struggle resulted that was resolved by the hospital comfort care committee.

General issues raised by this patient's plight include:

1. The fact is that many patients want to die at home, but few really are really encouraged or even allowed to do so in our current medical system.
2. Hospitals for most individuals have not only become a place of care delivery but also an arena for dying, as contrasted to dying in the familiar and meaningful

environment of home. Resources are not present for transitioning to a home death when assisted ventilation (life support) is involved.

3. The hospice model, with all its laudable features, does tend to support a hospital death for patients who are already in the hospital.
4. Significant medical costs are incurred in end-of-life care.
5. The decision to institute life support measures including tracheostomy for assisted ventilation, gastric tubes for provision of nutritional support, and aggressive surgeries in near-futile situations is almost always made in the moment of medical emergencies. Family considerations and patient directives are often lost at that point. Informed consent frequently is obtained under the duress of medical urgency.

These decisions must be undertaken with great caution and deliberation. The overwhelming attraction in patient management in critical, life-threatening circumstances is to do "more" when the "more" may be opposite of patient's wishes and even lead to a painful, even tormenting, demise.

Complexity Summary

1. Biological (including genetic)
   Acute:
   - Admitted to our local long-term acute care (LTAC) hospital with a methicillin-sensitive *Staphylococcus aureus* bacteremia and an infected abdominal aortic aneurysm discovered during endovascular repair (graft) for that aneurysm
   Chronic:
   - Ventilator dependence. Cardiovascular issues of congestive heart failure. Abdominal aortic aneurysm associated with peripheral vascular disease. Necrotic toes also likely associated with peripheral vascular disease. Persisting staphylococcal infection. Hospital-acquired *C. difficile* enteritis
2. Psychiatric/psychological
   - This is not possible to discern because of his altered level of consciousness during most of his hospital stay. At times he was minimally responsive to his environment. At best he was lethargic for periods of time; at other times he was stuporous and minimally responsive.
3. Social (including family and other support systems)
   - He was being taken care of by a neighbor who developed cancer during his hospital stay and could no long care for him. His grandson who lived at a distance was minimally available until the issue of where he would die was raised.
4. Care delivery, including access to care
   - The patient was dependent on care systems that had no personal contact with his family. His access to care was limited to our local LTAC.

5. Fundamental factors supporting or obstructing the treatment, in particular quality and continuity of the physician-patient relationship
   - Patient's inability to actively work with his provider made treatment an entirely unilateral process. When it came close to the end of his life, his grandson was obstructionistic with hospital staff, insisting that the patient be allowed to die at home (often desirable but inappropriate in this case). The final chapter of this saga is marked by the grandson and his attorney's problematic entry into this case (see reflections from author). Sadly, all involved were sympathetic to the idea of the patient's dying at home. Had there been more family available to support his option, perhaps it could have been accomplished.
   - Final issues governing this case were logistical (practical), i.e., managing the patient's demise at his home, and ethical, i.e., who should make decision about where and how a patient dies. As in this case, ethical considerations may be a major component of case complexity. Family-based disruptions, requiring major management adjustments, seriously threatened his care on several occasions. Quick and judicious action, as well as constancy by his PCP was required at several medically critical points to implement these actions and protect the patient and his treatment.

Chapter 23
Advance Care Planning for Patients with Current and Future Medical Complexity

Lael Duncan

The author traces the courses of two aging patients from physical health to death. She highlights the process of creating an advance care directive and Physician Orders for Life-Sustaining Treatment (POLST). These documents provide guides for patients' physicians in the event that lifesaving measures become necessary. Discussions needed to guide a patient through medical requirements as the end-of-life approaches are also illustrated.

Two patients are used for illustration. The first is Mr. T., a 62-year-old man with a history of myocardial infarction and class II heart failure. He also has history of diet-controlled type II diabetes mellitus. The second is Mrs. G., a 72-year-old widow with a history of chronic obstructive pulmonary disease (COPD) and osteoarthritis. She has a daughter age 43 with special needs who lives with her. Mrs. G. previously required breathing assistance and intubation. She will need a knee replacement, and understands that she may not be able to tolerate the operation. However, she is eager to sustain her life and not abandon her daughter. Months later she presented with increased cough, chest pain, and gradual weight loss. Additional studies revealed pulmonary, hepatic, and central nervous system metastatic disease. Non-small cell lung cancer was confirmed with biopsy.

The author takes us through years of the lives of these two patients, illustrating the development of their ultimately terminal systemic medical diseases. Highlighted is the management of the personal challenges that ensued as physicians guided preparation for their ultimate demise.

L. Duncan, MD (✉)
Internal Medicine, Coalition for Compassionate Care of California, Sacramento, CA, USA
e-mail: lael.md@gmail.com

© Springer International Publishing AG, part of Springer Nature 2018

S.A. Frankel, J.A. Bourgeois (eds.), *Integrated Care for Complex Patients*,
https://doi.org/10.1007/978-3-319-61214-0_23

"We are the benefactors and the victims of scientific success." Ira Byock, The Best Care Possible. A physician's quest to transform care through the end of life. (Avery 2013)

Introduction

The twentieth century ushered in unprecedented scientific advances that measurably improved our ability to care for patients with serious, complex, or advanced illness. These medical advances, along with increase in the population of persons aged over 65 years, have fostered an increase in the prevalence of serious chronic illness. Many of us will live longer than our predecessors, but with a greater overall burden of disease. To best manage the medical and psychiatric burdens of these patients, we need to ensure that the care we give is focused on patient-centered quality outcomes. An unfortunate circumstance of our complex medical system is that aggressive and occasionally routine ongoing care can be delivered without focusing on real wellness and patient-defined values. Physical dependence, dementia, and disability are now common occurrences in the last chapter of life for many patients. Survey data indicates that one quarter of 80-plus-year-olds are affected by neurocognitive disorder (NCD)/dementia, mostly moderate. Prevalence rates of dementia do not level off, but continue to rise gradually even in the extremes of age [1]. Most of these patients have additional medical problems, and many are patients with systemic medical-psychiatric comorbidities. These vulnerable populations deserve the opportunity to define and receive care that is focused on outcomes which they find meaningful.

If we are going to provide respectful, efficient, patient-centered, family-focused care for our aging population, we should implement strategies and systems that will address the complexities so often seen in the final stages of life. Patients and families can benefit from opportunities to plan for anticipated and unanticipated emergency events that may present complex options for care. Our current healthcare workforce and common healthcare practices, which focus on short- or long-term medically centered (physiologic, not patient-centered) outcomes, will be insufficient to meet patient needs [2]. Processes and systems that work to improve the overall value, efficiency, and cost-effectiveness of care for geriatric or medically complex patients should have wide appeal. Advance care planning is one of our better options for improving the quality of care delivered to patients in these populations.

Advance care planning is the process of communication among the patient, clinicians, family, and/or other individuals intended to clarify treatment preferences, identify a surrogate decision-maker, and develop goals for care in serious illness and near the end of life. The planning process is based on effective conversations and information exchange; documentation of key elements, is a critical component. Elements of the plan to be documented include individual goals and values, and the patient's perspective on how future decisions should be made if the patient is incapacitated. Any relevant legal or medical forms completed as part of the process should be entered into the medical record and shared with family members or surrogate decision-makers. The advance care planning process informs and supports patients and families facing complex choices or anticipating future healthcare decisions. Additional benefits include improved family satisfaction and reduced caregiver stress [3]. The goal of advance care planning is to align treatment choices with patient-centric value-based care preferences and to have that information available to providers and family when the need arises. Advance care planning is particularly important for patients of high medical complexity. High-complexity patients are usually faced with greater overall numbers of activities and treatments necessary to maintain health. Family and caregivers are under stress from the emotional, physical, and logistical burdens of caretaking for these patients [4]. Paradoxically, these complex patients are also especially vulnerable to overtreatment [5]. Achieving patient-centered care in this setting is a significant challenge. For patients with chronic, progressive, and/or complex disorders, advance care planning can assist with the alignment of short- and long-term goals—both physiologically and functionally based. Advance care planning discussions provide a framework in which treatment choices can be considered in order to help prepare families and healthcare agents for future, complex decisions.

Our youth-obsessed culture and our healthcare system—whose default is to always treat in the absence of an absolute contraindication—have not traditionally supported a role for advance care planning. With the advent of palliative care as a recognized (and now board certified) subspecialty and the rise of empowered, socially active, engaged patients, this tradition is changing. Mainstream media, which continues to saturate us with revolutionary ideas about the potential for human longevity, is now willing to pay more needed attention to our inevitable mortality and to the way end of life happens for patients, families, and clinicians.

The roots of this shift in focus can be traced back to the 1970s, when the first of several highly publicized legal cases raised public awareness about the need for legal surrogate healthcare decision-makers. Finally enacted in the wake of the United States Supreme Court's *Cruzan* decision in 1990, the Patient Self-Determination Act (PSDA) established a patient's right to autonomy with respect to lifesaving or life-prolonging care [6]. This legislation established the role and responsibilities of the surrogate medical decision-maker, the durable power of attorney for healthcare decisions, or medical durable power of attorney (other commonly used terms include: healthcare advocate, proxy, or agent).

Sadly, the documents intended to protect these rights and to assist and empower the surrogate decision-maker, "the advance (health/medical) directive and the living will" remain woefully underutilized, with only about 26% completion among all adults and 48% completion rates among older community-dwelling adults [7]. Even when available, the documents themselves have often proven to be less than useful for family members and often clinicians as well [8]. This situation may result when the named healthcare agent has not been directly informed by the owner of the document as to that person's care preferences. Families and clinicians often cannot fully know what treatment a patient wants when that patient is not able to speak for himself/herself.

There may be other related problems. Clinicians providing invasive or life-sustaining care to patients whose wishes are unknown may find making these decisions personally stressful. Burdensome decision-making can lead to emotional trauma for the family, in turn resulting in traumatic and stressor-related disorders among anxious family members [9]. By addressing these patients, family, caregiver, and provider needs, advance care planning systems can vastly improve our ability to achieve quality-focused patient-centered goals.

In addition to improving patient-centered outcomes, advance care planning helps health systems improve value in end-of-life care and secondarily may achieve significant savings by reducing overall undesired or non-beneficial hospitalizations or intensive care treatments [10, 11]. Thus, the implementation of effective advance care planning systems within the broader array of healthcare settings will enhance our ability to provide the best care possible in even the most challenging situations.

What follows in this chapter is a case-based description of effective advance care planning and recommendations for clinicians wishing to embrace these principles. The US Centers for Medicare and Medicaid Services (CMMS) now formally recognizes this work and with newly implemented CPT codes (99497, 99498) provides reimbursement for advance care planning. The time for advance care planning to become part of routine health has come.

A recent poll by the John Hartford Foundation [12] indicates that providers are often ill prepared to facilitate these discussions either because they have not been trained to do so, do not have staff to assist in the process, or do not have a way to record and track goals of care discussions. Processes, infrastructure, and training are needed to create sustainable advance care planning systems. Many healthcare organizations are now looking at ways to integrate advance care planning into routine care for target populations such as those with cancer and advanced heart, lung, or kidney disease or other populations with complex medical illness. Some are integrating advance care planning into routine healthcare for all patients, making it a normal, anticipated part of good medical care.

Elements of Advance Care Planning

There are three phases to advance care planning: exploration, expression, and implementation (when patient wishes are honored). Exploration of the kind of care a patient wants ideally begins in the home. Patients, possibly along with their family, friends, spiritual leaders, and/or community educators, can consider what values and beliefs they hold about life and health. They may need to think about what brings quality to their life and maximizes or defines "good health" for them. Personal reflection, consideration of a surrogate decision-maker, and learning about advance health directives are other initial steps in this exploration phase. Patients may also need to meet with clinicians during this phase to discuss individual treatment benefits and potential burdens. Depending on patient age, stage of disease, or urgency, this phase may be simple and short or complex and long.

Following this exploration, patients express their wishes and concerns to their family, their surrogate decision-maker, and their clinicians. Wishes or care preferences can then be documented in the medical record. An advance healthcare directive

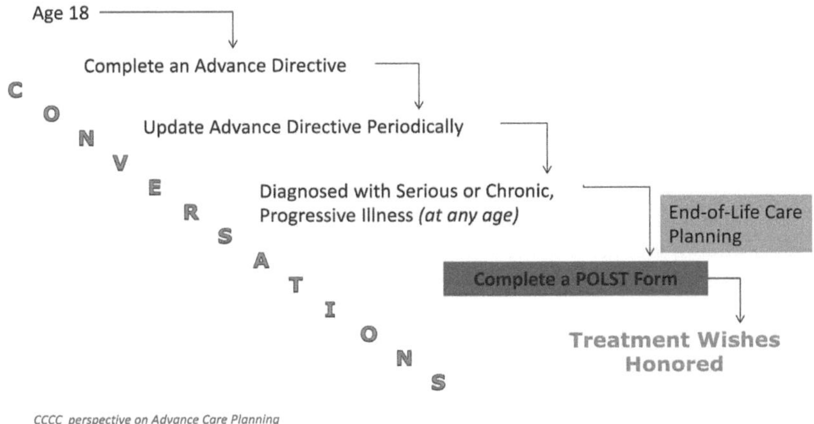

ACP Continuum, Duncan

(or advance medical directive), including appointment of a durable power of attorney for healthcare (DPOA-HC), should also be completed at this time. The advance healthcare directive document should be accessible to the named healthcare agent. Supporting documentation, which can take the form of a letter to family, voice recording, or video, can also be completed if desired.

Keeping conversations and documentation up-to-date is essential. Discussions are revisited over time and as circumstances change. As a good starting point, review and updating of conversations and documents should occur every 5 years in times of stable health. Significant health or life events should trigger a review of care plans. Such events should include new serious illnesses, anticipated surgery, and also changes in family structure (e.g., birth, death, divorce, family relocation). Updates and revision of any documents should occur on a regular basis keeping dates current and in a chronological manner that minimizes confusion. Upon completing updates, earlier versions of these documents should be clearly voided or destroyed.

In the event of a serious medical illness or accident, which renders the patient unable to speak for himself/herself, previously expressed wishes can be honored. The decisions should be reflective of the wishes and values the *patient* has previously expressed. Lastly, late in life, when health and vitality wane, advance care planning should involve a discussion of preferences for end-of-life care, including preferences for life-sustaining treatments and resuscitation. These challenging, often delicate discussions are most productive when done in the context of clarifying how a patient defines quality in his/her life and articulates his/her beliefs and values. Goals of care need to be both meaningful to the patient *and* medically acceptable to the health system. Discussion of resuscitation, intensive care, respiratory support, and artificial hydration and nutrition are usually required. When choices are made for or against resuscitation, it is imperative that this information is available to the decision-maker, family, and treating clinicians. Many states now use Physician Medical Orders for Life-Sustaining Treatment (POLST or MOLST) forms, for example. There are different versions of this form in different states.

POLST

Physician Orders for Life-Sustaining Treatment (POLST) is a unique transferable medical order form that gives seriously ill patients control over their end-of-life care. Included in POLST are medical treatment orders reflecting patient choices for or against intensive measures (such as the use of a ventilator or introduction of artificial nutrition) and cardiopulmonary resuscitation (CPR). Printed on brightly colored paper and signed by both a physician and the patient, POLST can prevent unwanted or non-beneficial treatments, guide clinicians toward desired treatments, and ensure that a patient's wishes are honored. By providing clarity around patient choices, use of these forms may reduce family/surrogate decision-maker distress. In states or regions where the form has legislative backing, it can constitute a valid medical order, accepted in community and healthcare settings. Information on POLST programs is available on the website of the National POLST Paradigm at www.POLST.org. Check this site for information on a POLST Paradigm program in your state.

The Conversation

The nuanced discussions and family meetings that result in actionable advance care planning documents, such as the patient's recorded goals of care, or a POSLT form, are often referred to as "Having *The Conversation.*" These conversations can occur in community or healthcare settings. Participants can include the patient, family members, primary care provider, and others such as a trained facilitator, caretaker, consulting physician(s), nurse, chaplain, psychologist, or social worker. Specifically, having "*The Conversation*" implies a discussion of the type of care the patient would want in the event of a serious illness when he/she is unable to advocate or speak for himself/herself at the end of life. *The Conversation* is the most critical element of the advance care planning process.

The Impact of Setting on Advance Care Planning Interventions

Outpatient Advance Care Planning

In the outpatient setting, initial activities of advance care planning include general discussions about health and risk and education about the purpose of the advance health directive or living will. The patient and family members learn how to choose an appropriate surrogate decision-maker and how to inform the chosen individual about their role and responsibilities and about the patient's preferred goals of care. Providers or advance care planning facilitators prompt, encourage, and assist patients and families to complete basic advance directives. Plans are revisited or revised as needed when there are changes in health status and/or family structure. For patients with serious chronic conditions, education is provided on the technicalities and possible outcomes of resuscitation and life support treatments. This part of the discussion should include asking the patient to describe unacceptable outcomes, states of health in which the patient might wish to choose comfort-focused care and forego life-prolonging measures.

Inpatient Advance Care Planning

Patients in hospitals, skilled nursing facilities, and other care settings need a surrogate decision-maker. Most often, the name of that person is obtained on admission. Supporting documentation such as an advance health directive should be included in the medical record, if available. Most facilities have forms to reflect preferred intensity of care and preferences on resuscitation. If a POLST form is available, it should be on file. Most critical for these patients is that their choices be appropriately reviewed and discussed with them and/or with the surrogate decision-maker at the time of admission or when there are changes in the patient's condition or prognosis. Acute and long-term risks with likely outcomes evolve as the patient's health status changes. Implicit at the time of admission to a hospital or other facility is the fact that the patient's health status is changing and review of care preferences is indicated. Such changes should prompt reconsideration and revision of goals of care. These discussions and any supporting documentation should be entered into the medical record and shared with the surrogate decision-maker.

Advance Care Planning and the Emergency Department

It is a distressing fact of the fractured US health system that most patients arrive at the emergency department without having had access to advance care planning. Frail elderly patients, critically ill patients, and those who are repeatedly admitted for the treatment of progressive conditions, such as congestive heart failure, late-stage pulmonary disease, major neurocognitive disorder (formerly dementia), and/or end-stage renal failure, present logistical, social, emotional, and financial challenges to the frontline clinicians and to the health system at large. In the absence of advance care planning, the goals of care for these patients are usually unclear. Without the guidance that care planning can provide, intensive life-prolonging care may be repeatedly administered, despite potentially poor short- and long-term outcomes. Often the patient and family are unaware of the potential outcomes and associated burdens, and they may request repeated interventions despite lack of alignment with the patient's goals for care. Without access to information that conveys the patient's wishes, the frontline clinicians struggle to provide guidance for families and decision makers. In settings where the staff are trained and have access to documentation that reflects the patient's goals of care and includes support from services such as palliative care or counselors to assist with care planning conversations, care planning can be accomplished even in the emergency setting.

Illustrative Clinical Scenarios

Scenario 1: Mr. T.

Mr. T. (a fictional composite patient) is a 62-year-old man with a history of myocardial infarction and class II heart failure. He has history of mild hypertension, diet-controlled type II diabetes mellitus, and trace proteinuria. He worked as an accountant and enjoyed golf, travel, and reading. He presented to his primary care physician, Dr. James, for a routine physical and medication review. Advance care planning activities for this stable middle-aged patient without prior advance care planning include education about how to choose a surrogate decision-maker and the importance of an advance healthcare directive. His clinician might also initiate a discussion about what type of care he would want in the event of an emergency.

After the physical examination was completed, Mr. T. says, "I read an article about long-term care and it got me thinking. How do I choose someone to speak for me if an emergency happens?" "I am glad you asked that today; I had hoped to talk to you about this during our visit," says Dr. James. "It is important to choose that person carefully. Often the first person we think of as a good choice is not going to be the right one. I can give you some guidelines for choosing a healthcare agent. Would that help you?" Mr. T. says "yes" and Dr. James goes on, "Ideally you want to pick someone with the following qualities: Your healthcare agent should be willing and able to be your spokesperson. He/she should be easily available, at least by phone. He or she should be well informed about your preferences and values and willing to speak in your voice despite their own feelings or preferences. This person should be comfortable making independent decisions and able to work with a medical team in potentially stressful conditions. Can you think of anyone who might fit that description?"

After careful thought and further discussion, Mr. T. choses one of his children, his son David, and the discussion continues. "It is important to let the rest of your family know who you have chosen and to choose a second person in case we cannot get hold of David right away. I am going to give you some resources that will guide you through the next part of this process as you think about your wishes and values. Then you can look at the advance healthcare directive and legally appoint David as your spokesperson along with your second choice. If you want to include some information about the kind of care you want, you may do that. I look forward to following up with you on this at our next visit."

For the next few years Mr. T. did well with medical therapy. His health profile was unchanged at age 67 and he remained active. He presented for a routine clinic visit with no new concerns and no new or progressive problems by physical exam and laboratory evaluation. At this time Dr. James says, "It seems like you are doing quite well. Some time has passed since we discussed your care planning. Let's review your choice of agent and any care preferences you have. I need to understand what is most important to you so we can have a care plan in place that works towards your current goals." They reviewed Dr. James' notes and David remained as the first healthcare agent along with Richard, the other son, as a second agent.

Dr. James asks, "Tell me what you know about CPR or cardiac resuscitation." Mr. T. replies, "Well, I know you can rescue a guy who is having a heart attack. I have seen it work on TV." A discussion ensues and includes patient education about the purpose and efficacy of CPR, particularly how it might apply in Mr. T.'s case since he already has significant heart disease. After this discussion, Mr. T. states he would want to receive CPR and intensive care if he had a sudden cardiac event. This information was recorded and shared with specialist clinicians who were likely to be involved if Mr. T. had a medical emergency. Dr. James concludes "It is very important that you discuss your choices along with your reasoning for those choices with David and Richard."

Change in Circumstances

Mr. T. is now aged 83. He has had two documented myocardial infarctions in the last 3 years and has undergone angioplasty on both occasions. Clinically he has advanced heart failure and progressive renal failure. Thus, he now has multiple risk factors for a sudden life-threatening event or death in the subsequent 6 months to a few years. He is seen in a follow-up visit after his most recent hospitalization. David is with him.

At this time, it is important for his clinicians to know more about his values and his perspectives regarding choices in care, specifically with respect to end-of-life care and life-sustaining treatments. What medical and personal issues is he most worried about? What kind of care could best help him through the days to come?

What about his life does he most enjoy? Are there medical situations he would find unacceptable such as loss of cognitive function and/or long-term ventilator dependence? Answers to such questions as these can help clinicians know how to prioritize and focus his care. With advance care planning at this stage, we can identify critical goals of care that will guide clinicians, the patient, and family members/surrogate decision-makers toward desired care and might allow for avoidance of unwanted treatments or unnecessary prolongation of suffering. Personal health goals can be translated into medical treatment plans. Ideally, a POLST form should specify patient preference for or against resuscitation and other life-prolonging treatments. Including healthcare agents and other family members in goals of care discussions is important.

After his medical examination and a discussion of his medication, his current clinician, Dr. Singh, says, "Mr. T., a lot has happened in the last year or two. You have had a few close calls. I want to be sure that if an emergency comes up we know how you want to be cared for. It is important to me to respect your values. Can we talk about this?" "Sure, but what do you mean?" "Well" (Dr. Singh goes on), "If your heart or kidneys stop working those would be very bad things. There is a chance that our usual treatments wouldn't work. I worry about that. I worry that we might try to treat you but that things might not go well. If that happens, I want to know how to help you best. Does that make sense?"

Mr. T. takes a deep breath. "Yes, they talked to me about this in the hospital last time, but I didn't really get it. They talked about the kidney machine. I think I was, maybe… scared. I worry about these things. My father didn't go out easy, know what I mean? That was tough. I don't want to go like that." Dr. Singh: "It sounds like your father's death was hard on you, maybe the family too. I am sorry to hear that. Can you tell me more?" "Well, my dad was sick for a long time, but the end seemed to drag on. He got a lot of treatment but I don't think it was making him better near the end and he seemed so miserable. Finally he just died in the hospital. No one was there. He had been really short of breath or something, and they couldn't fix it. I don't really know but when I think of that, it makes me sad… and angry." "It really does sound like that was tough." Both paused to reflect on this experience.

Then Dr. Singh continues. "Would you like to make some plans so that we understand how you would want to be treated as time goes by or if your health takes a turn for the worse? We can talk about what to do if our current treatments are not working well for you and outline the other types of treatment and care you would want at that time. I want to ensure that you are comfortable until the end of your life, whenever we face that. Would this help?" "Yes, I think I would sleep better if I knew that."

Dr. Singh and his staff spent time during the next few appointments working to understand what critical care treatment Mr. T. would want and when he would no longer want medical treatment to sustain his life. The basis for these choices, as a reflection of his values, was recorded. His sons were included in the discussions. Afterward, Mr. T. confirmed that he would want CPR and ICU care "if it works." He agreed that *trial periods* of intensive therapy are right for him. He completed a

POLST form indicating his preferences. Dr. Singh concluded, "I hope we don't have to face any of these events soon, but I am glad to know what is important to you and how to treat you best if something happens."

Although advance care planning encounters are challenging for patients, many will experience relief and a sense of comfort after a discussion of their fears and reassurance that physical symptoms such as pain and dyspnea can be managed. Some patients may wish to engage in planning for the last phase of life more actively by preparing their legal papers, finances, or belongings. Finding closure in key areas of life and relationships can offer a sense of peace in this last phase of life.

Reevaluation and Revision of Plans

At age 85, Mr. T. had severe refractory congestive heart failure and was hospitalized. He was not a candidate for mechanical circulatory support or surgical intervention. His advance healthcare directive and resuscitation choices were reviewed. During this admission, he had a potentially lethal arrhythmia. CPR was implemented and he responded to treatment after 12 min. He subsequently received care in the ICU including ventilator support and sedation. The medical team described his prognosis for meaningful recovery—as defined by the patient in prior discussion of choices and values— to be minimal. His cardiac rhythm remained unstable, and he was high risk for repeated cardiac arrest.

Should aggressive care be continued at this point? Should CPR be implemented in the event of another arrest? In most cases, the treatment preferences indicated on a POLST (or equivalent) form should be respected. However, there are other considerations. For example, changes in circumstances or changing patient values should prompt a reevaluation of the patient's choices and corresponding medical orders. Prior discussions and the patient's preference for "trial periods only" suggested that he wanted treatments that would be effective and expected to assist him in recovery to his baseline or other acceptable state of health. If it becomes clear the treatments are not effective, the physicians should not be afraid to conclude that the ongoing trial of intensive therapy is not helping him as hoped and to propose no further escalation of care or possibly withdrawal of intensive support or transition to comfort-focused care. In the case of Mr. T., a family conference was called and was attended by his sons and the care team. In light of his previously expressed wishes for a trial of therapy, his goals for care were reviewed. His sons understood from earlier discussions with their father that he had wanted to "give things a try" if a health crisis occured. But they knew also that he would not want ongoing life support or prolonged intensive care if he was not expeted to "regain independence of action and thought," and would be "hooked up to machines" for survival. Along with current estimates of prognosis, palliative care and hospice were discussed and symptom managment was reviewed. Plans were made for compassionate discontinuation of the ventilator. Mr. T. died peacefully about two hours after extubation, with family at the bedside.

Scenario 2: Mrs. G.

Mrs. G. (a fictional composite patient) is a 72-year-old widow with a history of chronic obstructive pulmonary disease (COPD) and osteoarthritis. She has an advance healthcare directive, and her oldest daughter, Sue, is her healthcare agent. Her younger daughter, Debra, aged 43 has special needs and lives with the patient. In association with COPD flares and bronchitis, Mrs. G. previously required breathing assistance by noninvasive positive pressure mask on two occasions and intubation on one occasion. In the past, she responded well to therapy and was easily weaned from external breathing support. Her last admission was 1 year ago. At that time, she updated her advance directive and stated that she would be willing to undergo intubation again. She has been ambivalent about receiving CPR. When she is not acutely ill, she is very active. She volunteers regularly for community events, takes art classes, and loves gardening. Her days are full and busy.

Over the last year, her right hip joint has deteriorated, and she can no longer walk without severe pain. A joint replacement is indicated. In anticipation of surgery, her primary clinician, Dr. Allino, discusses her advance care plan. "Do you have any questions about the surgical risks we have gone over?"

"I don't think so." Mrs. G. replied.

"It would help me to be certain we understand each other. Can you explain to me what you think the risks are?"

"Well, I think we agree the biggest risk is that my lungs could get bad or something else could happen and you might not get me off the ventilator. That would be a tough situation. For me that is a big risk but I can't walk well right now and I have to be able to get around to take care of my daughter. I really feel I have to give this a try. If something bad happens, I want to be treated. I want every chance to get back to being active, even if it takes a long time."

"It sounds like you have given this serious thought. What other questions do you have for me?"

"None right now."

Then Dr. Allino says, "Have you gone over all this with your older daughter, Sue? Does she know your wishes and preferences for care? Does she understand about the surgery?"

"Yes, I have kept her up to date."

"It sounds like you are ready then."

Mrs. G. places high value on regaining and maintaining physical independence, and she is willing to take on the risks of general anesthesia and surgery. Older patients with chronic illness need to review healthcare wishes more frequently than healthy middle-aged adults. Surgery is always an indication to review the advance healthcare directive and choice of surrogate decision-maker. Time should be given to a discussion of any risks associated with intervention that have the possibility of impacting quality of life.

Anticipating End of Life

Mrs. G. tolerated her surgery and returned home after a short rehabilitation. For the next 6 years, she was managed as an outpatient and remained active. She is now aged 78. Three weeks ago, she presented with increased cough, chest pain, gradual weight loss, and a recent fall. Workup showed a 2.5 cm mass in the right upper lobe. Additional studies revealed pulmonary, hepatic, and central nervous system metastatic disease. Non-small cell lung cancer was confirmed after biopsy. She was offered chemotherapy. Radiation treatment is under discussion. She is now in the office of her primary clinician. She has lost 14 pounds in 6 months; she feels tired, weak, and short of breath. Her daughter, Sue, is with her. Mrs. G. says she is worried about her younger daughter and she has fears about the future.

Respiratory failure, prolonged intubation, and death are significant risks now for this patient. Advance care planning at this time should include a discussion about acceptable risks and desired outcomes. This information will help her clinicians to understand how decisions should be made in the event that she becomes incapacitated. Including the healthcare agent in the conversation and documenting these discussions are critical to the success of her care plan. If a POLST form, or its equivalent, can be completed in advance, that will assist clinicians in the event of an emergency.

It is important to give Mrs. G. the opportunity to express her concerns about end of life and to discuss her thoughts about her quality of life. She may or may not be able to describe states of health that would be unacceptable to her. That is, she may be emotionally unprepared for that type of discussion. Additional conversations with Mrs. G. and her older daughter will be necessary as she gains understanding and acceptance of her condition.

Due to the sensitive and emotionally charged nature of these topics, patients vary widely in their ability to engage in productive end-of-life planning. Often there is a disconnection between what they logically or cognitively understand to be true and what they feel on an emotional level. For example, a patient may understand that a diagnosis is terminal yet unable to discuss the future. On some days, he or she may be ready to finalize a will or financial arrangements, but later that same day may be unable to discuss life-sustaining treatment. This could be, for example, because, on the one hand he or she understands (cognitively) that death is on the near horizon, but on the other (emotional), he or she cannot tolerate leaving behind a beloved family member. It is normal in this setting for patients to express ambivalence about resuscitation. Cognitive and emotional integration of a terminal diagnosis takes time and these processes can proceed at different rates. Sometimes several conversations are needed in order to make progress toward a plan for end-of-life care.

In some settings, an advance care planning facilitator, often a nurse or other clinician trained in advance care planning and end-of-life conversations, can spend the needed time with these patients. The primary clinician or specialist is then able to focus on treatment decisions and other tasks. Skilled clinicians can gather at least some critical information in this type of emotionally charged setting in as little as

6–15 min per visit, according to experts. Completing a full plan of care often takes more time.

Emergency Advance Care Planning and Palliative Care

Mrs. G. received whole-brain radiation and her CNS lesions receded. She began a difficult course of chemotherapy treatment, and at 8 weeks CT (computed tomography) and PET (positive emission tomography) scan evaluation indicated some improvement. Despite many discussions about treatment, quality of life, and prognosis, she had not been able to complete a POLST form or make a decision about a do-not-resuscitate order for herself. She regularly expressed concern and anxiety about how her daughter would be cared for in her absence.

At 10 weeks into treatment, she suffered further weight loss, fatigue, nausea, and progressive dyspnea (shortness of breath). Physical symptoms were making it difficult for her to care for her younger daughter at home. Chemotherapy was suspended to preserve quality of life, and over the next few weeks, she gained strength. She decided to forgo further treatment in order to avoid side effects. Six months later, she presented in respiratory distress with cachexia (wasting), anemia, and hepatic insufficiency. CT scan now showed growth of the previously noted lesions and new metastatic disease in the chest, abdomen, and brain. She was awake and speaking, but with difficulty. She appeared frail and tired. Her older daughter Sue was with her. She required urgent intubation to which she agreed. Discussion with the oncologist, pulmonologist, and ICU clinician indicated poor prognosis for recovery with or without treatment directed at the cancer.

Avoiding burdensome non-beneficial treatments is one goal of advance care planning. In this case, Mrs. G.'s earlier ambivalence about intensive care and resuscitation made her intubation in this setting inevitable. Ongoing intensive care in this situation cannot achieve an outcome with value for the patient. What she always wanted from her treatment, her goal, was to remain active and to retain the ability to care for an adult child with special needs. Her clinicians all agreed this was no longer an achievable goal. It was appropriate now for her treatment team to assist the patient and family with the transition from aggressive intervention to a care plan that anticipated end of life. At this point, the treatment team could sit with the patient and family and support them through a decision-making process.

Putting ACP to Work in Healthcare Settings

Implementation of successful advance care planning programs within healthcare organizations takes into account the need for careful planning, leadership, and administrative support. Essential components of a program include training for clinical and support staff, ongoing education, materials, electronic medical record processsing, and data tracking. Sensitivity to work flow and patient needs is also necessary. Community education and awareness activities that focus on advance care planning can support and dovetail with existing and emerging hospital or organizational programs.

Targeted endpoints for an advance care planning program include alignment of treatment plans with patient-centered medically acceptable goals and patient and family satisfaction with the care received. Collateral results include avoiding burdensome, non-beneficial treatments and reduction in per-patient costs at the end of life while maintaining care quality and satisfaction. The American College of Physicians, in a report in November 2014 [13], indicated that communications about goals of care in serious illness are included among the five "best low-cost, high-value healthcare interventions."

Reflection

Most of us went into medicine to help people who suffer from medical illness. We wanted to diagnose, treat, and cure, and as part of this to collaborate with colleagues to implement cutting-edge science. Presently, many of us find ourselves fighting for the time to have an adequate conversation with a patient. Office visits may amount to a screen full of check boxes and flags reminding us of externally defined "best practices." Writing prescriptions or tracking down test results is often a digital labyrinthine experience.

This situation has to change. How can we reinvent a crippled system when we are so busy managing it? As with many innovations brought about by a strong social imperative, the public will need to be involved in this effort. They will need to be our ally in the fight to reinfuse medical care with a healthy dose of *actual care*.

Many communities have embraced the idea of public engagement and education about advance care planning and preparation for end of life. Community groups in various settings are developing and implementing programs to inform the public about this issue. With improved awareness, conversations about goals of care and care planning document completion are becoming more common. More often, patients and families are ready to argue for care that fits their value system and meets their urgent needs. More people are prepared to discuss end-of-life choices and preferences for or against resuscitation and life-sustaining treatments. They meet in community classrooms, recreation centers, cafés, places of worship, and homes, and they want to be heard. Slowly our public is becoming aware that our aggressive medical system does not always serve their best interests, and they are finding out what they can do about it.

If we as healthcare providers can harness this energy and merge these activities with clinician-led efforts to create sustainable and effective advance care planning programs within healthcare systems, we will go a long way toward supporting our patients and changing the culture of end-of-life care. When we inevitably find ourselves on the other side of the curtain, wearing the patient gown, it would be nice to have a warm reception!

Complexity Summary

Case 1

1. Biological (including genetic)
   Acute:
   - At age 62/67, no acute illness; at age 83, recent MIs and renal failure; at age 85, severe CHF and an assortment of other chronic diseases develop over approximately 15 years
   Chronic:
   - CAD/CHF, HTN, DM, renal failure
2. Psychiatric/psychological
   - No clear psychiatric illness, although at high risk for vascular dementia and delirium. As such, surveillance of decisional capacity is needed.
3. Social (including family and other support systems):
   - Employed until age 70, then retired, supported by family, housed, adequate social resources. Highly integrated family was of relevance in his avoiding psychiatric disorders associated with chronic medical decline, e.g., neurocognitive disorder (dementia), delirium, anxiety, and depressive disorders
4. Care delivery, including access to care
   - Adequately insured, good access to PCP and specialty care as needed. Physicians provide excellent personal support and explanation of medical condition and prognosis to patient
5. Fundamental factors supporting or obstructing the treatment, in particular quality and continuity of the physician-patient relationship.
   - The working relationships were based on mutual respect and trust of the physicians involved.
   - Functional ongoing PCP relationship. Trust of both providers was quite good.

Case 2

1. Biological (including genetic)
   Acute:
   - Age 72, bronchitis; age 78, metastatic cancer
   Chronic:
   - COPD, DJD
2. Psychiatric/psychological
   - No psychiatric illness initially. With cancer metastatic to the CNS, there is a high risk of neurocognitive disorder (dementia) and delirium. As such, surveillance of decisional capacity was needed. Of additional relevance is the patient's ever-present need to minimize the implications of her medical condition based on her need to care for her impaired daughter. She was therefore slow to embrace prophylactic or current treatment-related steps including the creation of an advance care plan. Perhaps hope and denial are implicated

factors, not necessarily pathological in themselves, but ultimately problematic for healthcare in situations like the present one.

3. Social (including family and other support systems)
   - Retired, stably housed, special needs daughter, supported by other family members, housed, adequate social resources
4. Care delivery, including access to care
   - Adequately insured, good access to PCP and specialty care as needed
5. Fundamental factors supporting or obstructing the treatment, in particular quality and continuity of the physician-patient relationship
   - While ostensibly committed to an ongoing PCP relationship, the patient repeatedly hesitated about completing her advance directives and was prone (for urgent personal reasons) to being self-willed about medical decisions. These tendencies impeded the healthcare she received especially at the termination of her life.

References

1. Lucca U, et al. Prevalence of dementia in the oldest old: the Monzino 80-plus population based study. Alzheimers Dement. 2015;11(3):258–70.e3.
2. Keehan SP, et al. National Health Expenditure Projections, 2016–25: Price Increases, Aging Push Sector To 20 Percent Of Economy. Health Affairs Mar 2017;36(3):553–63 doi 10.1377/hlthaff.2016.1627
3. Houben CH, et al. Efficacy of advance care planning: a systematic review and meta-analysis. J Am Med Dir Assoc. 2014;15(7):477–89.
4. Sautter JM, et al. Caregiver experience during advanced chronic illness and last year of life. J Am Geriatr Soc. 2014;62(6):1082–90.
5. Morgan DJ, et al. Setting a research agenda for medical overuse. BMJ. 2015;351:h4534.
6. Pope TM. Legal briefing: the new patient self-determination act. J Clin Ethics. 2013;24(2):156–67.
7. Rao, J. K., et al. Completion of advance directives among U.S. consumers. 2014 Am J Prev Med 46(1): 65–70. doi 10.1016/j.amepre.2013.09.008
8. Teno J, et al. Advance directives for seriously ill hospitalized patients: effectiveness with the patient self-determination act and the SUPPORT intervention. SUPPORT investigators. Study to understand prognoses and preferences for outcomes and risks of treatment. J Am Geriatr Soc. 1997;45(4):500–7.
9. Wright AA, et al. Associations between end-of-life discussions, patient mental health, medical care near death, and caregiver bereavement adjustment. JAMA. 2008;300(14):1665–73.
10. Zhang B, et al. Health care costs in the last week of life: associations with end-of-life conversations. Arch Intern Med. 2009;169(5):480–8.
11. Klingler C, In der Schmitten J, Marckmann G. Does facilitated advance care planning reduce the costs of care near the end of life? Systematic review and ethical considerations. Palliat Med. 2016;30(5):423–33.
12. National Poll - "Conversation Stopper: What's Preventing Physicians From Talking With Patients About End-Of-Life and Advance Care Planning?"http://www.johnahartford.org/newsroom/view/advance-care-planning-poll
13. Bernacki RE, Block SD. Communication about serious illness care goals: a review and synthesis of best practices. JAMA Intern Med. 2014;174(12):1994–2003.

Recommended Resources for Facilitating Conversations in Advance Care Planning and End-of-Life Care Choices

Back A, Arnold R, Tulsky J. Mastering communications with seriously ill patients: balancing honesty with hope. Cambridge, Cambridge University Press 2009.

R Buckman How to break bad news: a guide for health professionals. Baltimore Johns Hopkins University Press 1992.

Lo B. Resolving ethical dilemmas. A guide for clinicians. 5th ed. Philadelphia: Lippincott Williams & Wilkins; 2013.

Advance care planning and conversation resources for patients and clinicians are available at many online locations including the Coalition for Compassionate Care of California (CoalitionCCC. org), the website for the National POLST Paradigm (POLST.org), the National Hospice and Palliative Care Organization (NHPCO.org).

Suggested Additional Reading

Butler K. Knocking on Heaven's door: the path to a better way of death. Scribner reprint ed; 2014.

Gawande A. Being mortal: medicine and what matters in the end. New York: Metropolitan Books; 2014.

Kalanitihi P. When breath becomes air. New York: Random House; 2016.

Volandes A. The conversation: a revolutionary plan for end of life care. Paperback ed. New York: Bloomsbury; 2016.

Zitter, JN. Extreme Measures. Finding a Better Path to the End of Life. 2017 Avery, 1st Ed. ISBN-13: 978-1101982556

Chapter 24
Narrative Analysis of Complex Patient–Clinician Interaction from Our Sample

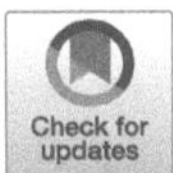

Carla Graf and Gina Intinarelli

Introduction

Clinically complex patients characteristically experience multiple physical and mental health challenges that lead to disability. They tend to have high health system utilization, may have poor social support, and lack adequate financial resources [1]. These patients tend to access healthcare providers and the health system repeatedly. Providers often do not have the requisite skill set to manage this range of complexity, and the health system may not support the full spectrum of patient needs, including access to specialty care or care coordination services. An integrated information system may also be missing.

As the understanding of the challenges of clinical complexity has evolved from medical diseases and complicated treatment plans alone, specialized assessment instruments have been developed to help providers identify patients at risk. Included are the INTERMED Complexity Assessment Grid [2] and the Minnesota Complexity Assessment Method [3]. These instruments incorporate mental health diagnoses, social determinants of health, patient engagement, and the availability of the health system itself. These critical patient factors must be assessed and addressed to guard against a patient with relatively straightforward diagnoses becoming a complex patient.

The linchpin for care of complex patients are primary care providers (PCPs) and specialists. A recent qualitative study of PCPs in academic and community settings

C. Graf, PhD, RN, GCNS (✉)
Office of Population Health and Accountable Care, San Francisco, CA, USA
e-mail: Carla.Graf@ucsf.edu

G. Intinarelli, RN MS PhD
University of California School of Nursing Social and Behavioral Sciences,
Vice President Department of Population Health University of California,
School of Medicine, San Francisco, CA, USA

Office of Population Health and Accountable Care, San Francisco, CA, USA
e-mail: Gina.Intinarelli@ucsf.edu

© Springer International Publishing AG, part of Springer Nature 2018
S.A. Frankel, J.A. Bourgeois (eds.), *Integrated Care for Complex Patients*,
https://doi.org/10.1007/978-3-319-61214-0_24

seeking to understand how PCPs conceptualize patient complexity resulted in a typology of complex patients in primary care [4]. This typology includes: "(1) medical complexity including discordant conditions, chronic pain, medication intolerance, unexplained symptoms, and cognitive impairment; (2) socioeconomic factors that exacerbate medical conditions: family stressors, inability to afford medications and transportation, and poor health literacy; (3) psychiatric illness exacerbating systemic medical conditions, e.g., depressive disorders, addiction, and anxiety disorders confusing the clinical picture; and (4) patient behaviors and traits, e.g., demanding of tests and medications, being argumentative with the clinical team, anxiety regarding symptoms" ([4], p. 452). One of the quotes from this study stated that a complex patient "is one who makes me think [about the patient when I am] outside of the exam room..." (p. 453). This quote became especially poignant to us as we reviewed our provider's narratives.

In this analysis, we offer further refinement of the factors previously described in the literature, especially noting the interplay between them as they affect patient outcomes and provider strategies for care.

Narrative Analysis Methodology

Narratives are a form of discourse that allows the participant to retrospectively organize and give meaning to a phenomenon or experience. Narrative is a way of organizing events into a meaningful whole while allowing the narrator to reflect upon the consequences of action over time. The narrator can communicate his/her point of view and include analytical reflections, interpretations, and emotions [5].

The interpreter seeks to identify the everyday reasoning or associations made by the participants through a systematic process of moving between the whole text and then to specific parts of the text. This process enables the interpreter to uncover incongruences or "unifying reported concerns" ([6], p. 113).

For this project, narratives of clinicians describing the everyday challenges and the practice of managing complex patients were analyzed for common themes, strategies, structures, processes, and congruencies. Health-focused narratives reveal health systems, patient and clinician factors that contribute to the various levels of challenge, and patient outcomes when caring for patients with complex syndromes. Articulating these factors enables caregivers and providers to adapt strategies to account for any deficiencies in these areas.

The basis of this chapter is an interpretive narrative analysis of 16 narratives written by community-based physicians, including primary care physicians, pediatricians, psychiatrists, neurologists, and sleep and pain specialists. The providers were asked to reflect upon and write about complex cases they had been involved with. The narratives include adult, adolescent, or pediatric patients with one or more complex illnesses. The majority of adult patients had more than one comorbid condition, including diabetes mellitus, cardiovascular disease, pain syndromes, and stroke. Most had diagnosed or suspected mental illnesses, and/or substance abuse; sometimes identified quite far into the care trajectory. Depression and anxiety were common; cognitive impairment, personality disorder, panic disorder, and anorexia nervosa were also present. These illnesses were often chronic and may have persisted throughout the patient's life. Chronic pain was associated with increased risk for substance use disorder in two of the cases. Pediatric and adolescent cases had a myriad of systemic medical illnesses as well, including allergies and nutritional problems, anorexia nervosa, ADHD, seizure disorder, post-viral encephalitis, and spinal cord injury. Mental health issues included drug dependence, opioid addition, oversensitivity to pain, and Munchausen syndrome by proxy.

Narrative and thematic analyses were conducted by two PhD nurses specializing in qualitative research methods. They also lead complex care management teams in an academic medical center. The text of these narratives was coded for themes in a qualitative software platform (Atlas, Ti); codes were examined and clustered into patient, system, and provider factors. Reflexive discussions of emerging themes were analyzed further with two psychiatry colleagues who are experts in complex care management. The analyzed text comprised 68 pages of extracted text and represented broad inclusive portions of the provider narratives.

Results

Patient, provider, and health system factors revealed several themes. Prominent patient factors were social support, resource availability, and "engagement capacity." Outstanding system and provider factors were the ability to create and sustain therapeutic and collaborative alliances and provider ability to discern and assess patient factors. Each theme was examined in depth with supportive text.

Provider and Health System Factors

Therapeutic Alliance

These narratives describe how complex patients were cared for by an "anchoring provider." We use this term to describe the provider who assumes the bulk of the patient care management and care coordination, sometimes fulfilling this role for years. While the primary care physician is often the anchoring provider, as evidenced by the narratives, this role may fall to any provider. For example, a pain specialist described how he assumed many roles in taking care of a very complex patient with "complex regional pain syndrome" [CPRS] and depression:

> *Mr. T.'s primary care physician started to work through a series of medications in an attempt to stabilize his pain. However, the county primary care clinic was inadequately equipped to provide the broad range of services necessary for management of Mr. T.'s CPRS…he eventually, with my help, transferred to a different regional clinic with the objective of achieving county sponsored housing*

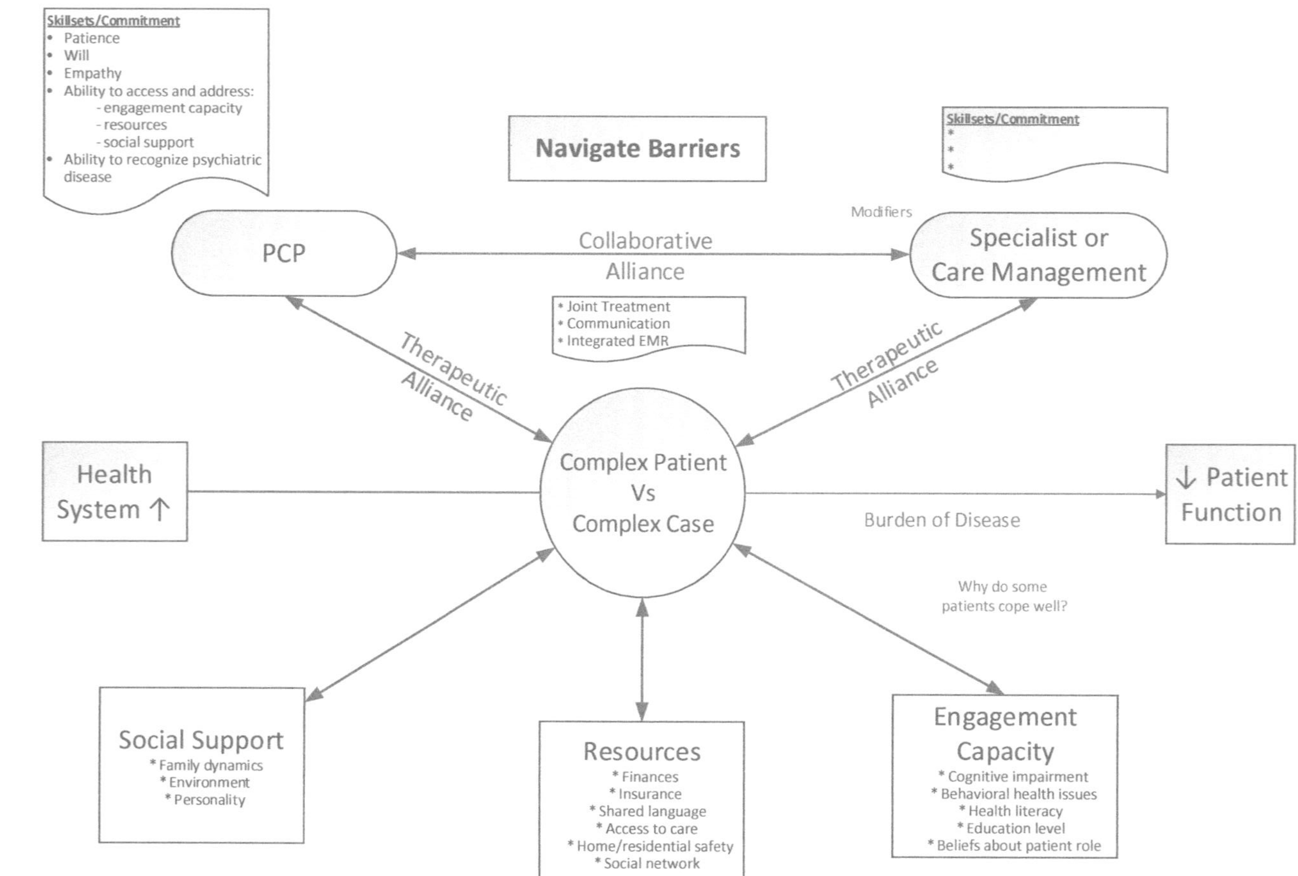

Navigating Barriers Visio Draft 1

Clinicians describe the importance of establishing and maintaining a therapeutic alliance with patients. They describe how they overcome barriers to creating an alliance which incorporates elements of trust, engaging conversations, and requires meeting the patient at his or her level. Many of the providers describe how they came to care for specific patients despite knowing the difficulty cases like this would cause them personally. Providers recognized the excessive time and effort it would take to care for this particular type of complex patient. Often the providers revealed that their motivation for creating and sustaining the connection to the patient involved feelings about the patient personally or that they admired the patient's intellect, creativity, or background. There was often a subtle acknowledgement of why they "clicked" or engaged with a given patient. For example, one provider recounted some the reasons he liked his patient, an adolescent patient with a severe substance abuse disorder:

> I liked her and found her intelligent, and was intrigued by her childlike inquisitiveness. I enjoyed discussing her experiences with meditation and existential philosophy and Buddhism

Others connected with patients on an intellectual level and established therapeutic alliance by engaging in interesting discourse and discussion as recounted by a psychiatrist who was treating a severely depressed man:

> John liked to debate epistemology, rationalism and empiricism

Yet, another physician expressed admiration for the way a young patient faced up to the reality of being a quadriplegic:

> Although he was aware that I already knew a lot about his story, Roger went on to describe how he ended up in a wheelchair...his seeming maturity and his ability to cope with his current state are what first struck me

Providers often had to lower their expectations about the type of gains they can make in forming a therapeutic alliance with patients who have limited engagement capacity; the providers often using slow and deliberate strategies to establish trust and a foundational relationship before they can make treatment recommendations. While they might have wanted to address the patient's urgent medical needs, they fear moving too quickly could "break" the therapeutic relationship so that at times they must:

> Play along, not challenging the patient for the purpose of sustaining a working relationship...this is appropriate when attempting to engage a resistant patient to comply with medical treatment

When the therapeutic alliance does not develop, including when patient attitude or behavior interferes with the work with collaborating providers, the patient may be at risk for being "fired" or ignored and the patient is likely to be labeled difficult and manipulative or hostile. This often occurs when undiagnosed or suspected psychiatric disease is present. When an alliance does not form with an "anchor" provider, complex patients are often tossed about like a hot potato, and referred to a series of providers, clinics, and other institutions. In many of the narratives, providers had to manage the failed relationships between the patient and other providers, often recognizing the patient's challenging behaviors as a key factor in these failures:

> *The pain and associated psychiatric manifestations increased and affected his relationships with other clinical providers. His affective lability, in the form of tearful frustrations… at times turned into angry outbursts…there was agreeing opinion that Mr. T was being manipulative*

The therapeutic relationship requires the clinician to go "above and beyond," working outside of the normal ways that he/she interacts with patients. They comment on the toll these relationships take on them and their staff, but yet they remain committed for years and remain willing to engage with these often time-consuming and difficult patient relationships. The providers recognize the difficulty and personal sacrifice they often are required to make when caring for these complex patients and the lasting impact these patients may have on them and their staff. As one provider recounts after one of their patients committed suicide:

> *It is impossible not to take some blame for MW's death, why MW stopped complying with our assessments and treatments is a mystery that will always haunt me. His picture still hangs in the clinic…for each patient you lose, a piece of your soul goes with them*

Providers who form a therapeutic alliance with their complex patients have often invested significant time, sometimes years into their treatment, may be left feeling incomplete with the outcomes. For example, one specialist described how after several years of treating two brothers for a set of complex neurological symptoms, the relationship was terminated abruptly. He was convinced that he understood their medical needs and had more to offer the patient:

> *At this point my involvement in S's care ceased. My role was that of the consultant and I was not invited to have a more general role in treatment. Equally, except for making suggestions, I was not successful in introducing appropriate specialists into his care, including mental health professionals…J's case suffered the same fate as that of his brother S, after the initial rounds of consultation, he disappeared from my practice…*

Ability to Assess and Manage Patient Factors:

It is clear that caring for a complex patient requires an expanded skill set for the anchoring provider, especially when there is a need to create a productive therapeutic relationship/alliance. The skills require include patience, will, empathy and the ability to assess and address three critical patient factors: engagement capacity, resources, and social support. The importance of this skill set cannot be underestimated. The "traditional" medical model does not place significant emphasis on the need to understand the patient's environment, in effect restricting the clinician's ability to thoroughly assess or act upon these factors. There can be significant barriers to fully understanding and mitigating any deficits in these three patient factor areas, as social support, engagement capacity, and resource needs are often not fully appreciated or recognized in traditional health care settings.

The ability to assess patient social support, resources, and engagement capacity often depends on access to family and friends in order to flesh out a complete picture of the patient's environment. In many cases, patients may guard against their healthcare providers learning about their lives "outside of the office." For example, a young woman insisted on "absolute confidentiality" which the provider recognized as a barrier to being able to treat her adequately. He reported feeling that he was:

> *Cut off from other sources of information that might inform my evaluation, forced to depend on an unreliable historian…my initial posture was directed at building a therapeutic alliance despite the chaos in her life. I rescheduled missed appointments and confronted her with her denials and the contradictions*

In another case, the clinician had assessed the significant family stressors that he felt contributed to the exacerbation of the patient's psychiatric disease and coping mechanisms:

> *The patient and family brought with them many social stressors to this hospital stay including a recent divorce, chronic illness, recent surgery for the patient's mother, a new diagnosis of autism for the patient's sibling and a diagnosis of cancer for the mother's boyfriend*

Ability to Recognize Psychiatric Disease:

A key skill for the anchoring provider is to always keep open the possibility of a psychiatric diagnosis. Frequently expressions of psychiatric disease are manifest as chaos in the patient's life or their interactions with the clinical providers and staff. These patients often present as manipulative, "non-adherent," and cause significant frustration to health care staff; they are time-consuming for all involved. The provider must further assess for the presence of psychiatric disease when there is social isolation, family estrangement, and/or manipulative behaviors. Some patients described in these narratives who had undiagnosed psychiatric disease were subjected to extensive medical tests to rule out "somatic" disease. Others were unable to form therapeutic alliances with their clinicians because of their reduced capacity to engage in meaningful relationships (e.g., due to depression, personality disorders, paranoia, and mistrust), resulting in fragmented care and poor outcomes. Upon reflection, several providers recognized the missed opportunity to address undiagnosed or suspected psychiatric disease. In an unusual case, a 6-foot tall woman, weighing only 90 pounds, was admitted to the hospital with advanced malnutrition, and while psychiatric disease was suspected, the patient still underwent significant medical testing to rule out nonpsychiatric causes before a diagnosis of anorexia nervosa was finally made by a psychiatrist.

> *The likely underlying cause was unconfirmed anorexia nervosa with possibly underlying depression exacerbated by hypothyroidism. However, given that there was no prior diagnosis of an eating disorder a more complete work-up was needed*

In another case, the physician reflected on the probability of psychiatric disease as a component after caring for two brothers with similar confounding symptomatology:

> *What does seem likely, however, is that in addition to systemic medical illnesses there was likely a major psychiatric component to the boys' presenting illness. This component was never formerly diagnosed or addressed*

Patients who have complex disease with a psychiatric component often do not get relief from traditional medical management and despite a myriad of tests and treatment regimens they remain in pain or suffer personally. They may lose trust with the health care system and are passed around to different specialists in search of a diagnosis. For example, in this case, the young man had been evaluated for several somatic complaints of pain in his neck and back, was evaluated with extensive diagnostic tests, but remained with no findings:

> *Tension at home was at a peak, leading Timothy in frustration, to throw a bottle of pills at his mother crying, "no one knows how to help me."*

Collaborative Alliance:

The ability to work collaboratively between the anchoring provider, other healthcare providers, and health systems is the key to the successful management of complex patients; the challenges to coordinate care and manage therapeutic collaborative relationships often fall to the "anchoring provider." Factors that promote a robust collaborative alliance can include agreement on diagnoses and treatment plans, collaborating to make a diagnosis, shared medical records, adequate communication patterns, and entrée/access to needed resources and facilities. Factors that inhibit collaborative alliance are a lack of a shared medical record, operating in different care delivery systems, a multiplicity of providers and/or disagreement on treatment plans, and/or splitting behaviors that may be introduced by the patient.

Breakdown of the collaborative alliance can introduce "iatrogenic complexity," for example, when two providers are at odds with treatment plans causing confusion and an increased complexity. In one example, the neurologist and the psychiatrist believe that a nasogastric tube for enteral feeding was a warranted potentially lifesaving measure for a delusional woman with severe malnutrition and anorexia nervosa; however, the hospitalist team disagreed and the patient remained in limbo for more than a week, before a feeding tube was eventually placed.

> *The hospitalist, however, cancelled the order feeling that the patient could not be mandated to eat and had a right to refuse artificial nutrition…eventually, a hospital ethics consult was obtained and determined the patient has severe mental illness, and was not decisionally competent*

Providers commented on the difficulty of operating in a fragmented health care system where "inter-clinician" communication and health system access are inhibited. They were unable to obtain critical information or unable to access the health systems; often, referral to a tertiary or quaternary health system offered little insight or advice on how to enhance the patient's treatment plans, as one provider explained:

> *Referrals were made to tertiary care centers for consultation or other assistance but the patient was repeatedly rejected for their services*

In one case, the deterioration of the therapeutic alliance between the patient and his mental health team, due to the patient's manipulative behaviors, required the relationship to be actively managed by the patient's "anchoring provider." The pain specialist recounts the strategies he used to soothe ruffled feathers and maintain the mental health care access the patient needed. He had to act as the "release valve" between the patient and his other providers using sophisticated strategies such:

Maintaining rapport with the patient, continually validating his frustration and concern while he simultaneously validated the concerns of the mental health providers as well, reviewing the 'contradictory evidence' about the patient's medical conditions, while validating all of their observations had merit

Providers recognize not only the importance of their "dedication to the patient and continuity of care" but also the "forbearance" required to manage these patients, often picking up the pieces from other treatments and/or searching for providers to help collaborate in the patient's care. For example, in one case, a long-standing patient was descending into chaos (e.g., estranged family, loss of home, and firing from an outpatient day center); she had also lost her long-standing psychiatrist and was having suicidal ideation. The primary care provider recounts on how she persisted in trying to find another psychiatrist who would accept her:

She began missing appointments with Dr. W and reported that he would not return her calls. He would not return my calls. Her social worker and I again looked at inpatient psychiatric units and alternate psychiatrists but were unable to locate any. We ultimately found a psychologist, Dr. K, who began seeing her.

There is a delicate interrelationship of all these factors, and the mitigation of deficits in any of these areas can significantly improve outcome. Two patients with the same comorbid medical conditions may have significantly different outcomes because of the presence or absence of these critical factors.

Patient Factors

Patient Chaos:

Patients identified as complex by providers often live "chaotic" lives, meaning that they have a myriad of medical, social, and behavioral problems that interfere with medical treatments as well as potentially interfering with the patient/provider therapeutic alliance. Chaos can affect access to resources, social support, and ability to engage with the healthcare team. Patients may live in chaotic situation. The chaos may result in homelessness and financial struggles, addiction issues, and loss of social support. Patients may not be able to engage in self-care until the chaos is mitigated. The health system or providers' practices may not have the resources available to both assess for and manage the contributing factors to chaos, such as psychiatric illness and social work services. Providers may struggle to prioritize the issues that need to be addressed, frequently relying on the medical model of treating an illness versus recognizing the underlying chaos that must be assessed and managed. In this example, the provider recounts how his patient, a university professor, quit his job due to mental health issues:

> *He was eager to talk and recounted his confused state of mind at the time he quit his professorship. In retrospect, he felt humiliated progressively realizing all that he had impulsively "thrown away."*

Patient chaos due to psychiatric disease affects many aspects of a person's life. MW's physical and mental illnesses were not only affecting his employment but his marriage was suffering as well:

> *As we talked it became clear that he had led a very productive early life that included many hobbies… A software engineer by trade he had fallen on hard times, however. When I met him he was feeling "hopeless," had trouble sleeping, snored endlessly and woke frequently with headaches. He complained of "lowness" and "lack of focus". He had arrived at a point where he could not finish a single project. These states of mind had affected his marriage and work and he was currently unemployed.*

Patients experiencing significant chaos may turn to their provider for assistance not only in treating their medical concerns but also in effect to become their case managers and social supports as illustrated by the narrative of Mr. T. Mr. T. experienced a long-standing chronic pain from an accidental knife injury. Mr. T's injury, and subsequent pain, treatment regimen and depression led to dropping out of business school, significant debt, and homelessness. As Mr. T was treated for his pain, his psychiatric manifestations intensified, his provider attempted to "facilitate transfer to a different regional clinic with the goal of achieving eligibility for county sponsored housing, close to a desirable tertiary care center":

> *The patient's personal and social situation had become tenuous. At this point, the patient was homeless and living in shelters. He was unable to attend school because of his disability and had lost all incoming money from his student loans. With worsening pain his ability to cope with the day-to-day struggles from a chronic medical condition and difficult psychosocial circumstances had worn thin …his pain, stress, and anxiety became manifest as sleep disturbance, fatigue, affective instability and frustration. His relationships with other clinicians were eroded.*

Patient chaos can occur when there is alignment of patient medical or psychiatric issues occurring at a time of lack of resources and/or poor social support. This situation is illustrated by the case of a 53-year-old woman admitted to the hospital with severe malnutrition and altered mental status due to anorexia nervosa. The chaos was perpetuated by little family support as her only advocate, her sister, out of frustration, resigned from the case. Case management was unable to place her in an eating disorders program due to insurance coverage issues. Previous to her admitting illness, she experienced an "anchoring event" with the death of a parent:

> *About 14 years previously, the patient's father died and the sister reported that the patient "went to pieces" afterwards. Their mother suffered from dementia and eventually was placed in a board and care facility. Their sister reported that the patient also had a great deal of difficulty dealing with her mother's decline.*

Subsequently, this patient experienced the consequences of alcohol abuse that led to arrest and loss of reliable transportation:

According to the sister the patient had a long standing history of alcohol abuse. At about age 50 and perhaps earlier the patient had a DUI arrest. She lost her license to drive and started bicycling to work. The patient (who was clearly not a reliable historian) reported that she has not had any alcohol since her arrest. She said she attempted to regain her driver's license but claimed that she failed "because of the cost."

Patient chaos is again illustrated in a case of an older woman followed for many years by her provider. This patient was estranged from most family members. Over time she persisted in utilizing the Emergency Department for care, calling 911 and incurring significant ambulance fees, depleting her modest finances, and making stable housing impossible. She hired and fired attendants, leading to difficulty in assessing her living situation, nutrition, and medication adherence. She had a history of emotional and physical abuse in her past with "evidence of borderline personality disorder, anorexia nervosa, relational dysfunction, substance abuse, somatization behavior, and a passive-aggressive approach to her own care":

She indicated a life long history of depression beginning in a difficult childhood. Her father was an alcoholic and her mother had severe mental health problems, possible schizophrenia. She had suffered physical, verbal, and probably sexual abuse.

She intermittently had a hired aide for one or two days a week and a hired financial planner took over bill paying. She was running out of money and clearly needing more help. Many of her caregivers suggested a move to an assisted living facility. She reported that Dr. W. was telling her to stay in her home and get a new tenant. Her daughter at this point was completely estranged and refused to help find a new tenant. She agreed to look at several facilities but after six months had not done so.

The chaos permeated middle age into older adulthood

She sold her house and moved to an assisted living facility. She was able to have an aide again 2 days/week. She developed bizarre eating habits-eating a single food for weeks at a time (crab salad or whipped cream). She would often only eat if her aide brought food to her. She started worrying about being "too fat" as her weight dropped to 112 pounds by August 2005. In 2006, she was evicted for continuing to smoke. She started a fire in a waste-basket with a discarded cigarette.

Resources:

Research has demonstrated that a lack of social and personal resources in addition to the stresses of *multimorbidity* can lead to coping difficulties for patients [7]. This may lead to decreased engagement and poor self-care. Resources, or lack thereof, are also cited by primary care providers as a common finding with the patients they identify as complex [4]. Problems with resources can include financial constraints, lack of access to care geographically, lack of or restricted insurance, lack of a shared language with providers, lack of home/residential safety, or lack of social networks. Having a lack of resources may create more work for the provider and teams as they try to implement a comprehensive care plan for their complex patients.

The following narratives demonstrate the difficulty the providers and patients experienced when trying to access psychiatric care when clearly a need existed:

> *Mrs. F had a difficult and long-standing depression which was resistant to many treatments. She did best with intensive 1:1 social support but cost and availability was frequently a challenge.*

> *By three weeks the patient had lost 2 additional pounds from her admission weight and remained limited in being able to comprehend her situation. Attempts to get her to an inpatient anorexia psychiatry program were unsuccessful do to insurance.*

> *One clinic in his town, a nearby town (30 miles) that has several specialties, and other primary care providers, one hospital. No psychiatrist within 75 miles. These logistical barriers to convenient care by specialists may have affected clinical outcomes.*

> *She began running out of medication and presenting in the office in opiate withdrawal. Her weight dropped to 126 pounds as she also reported having difficulty finding anything she wanted or could eat. She was hospitalized again with rapid heartbeat and an attempt to find an inpatient psychiatric unit to take her was unsuccessful.*

Having access to resources can improve patient outcomes as well as reduce the stress of the provider and the social supports. This is described by the provider of an older adult man with heart failure whose wife, at one time struggling as his primary caregiver, was also diagnosed with a significant medical illness:

> *Now, both the patient and his wife are cared for at home with full time caregivers and their two children are working together to coordinate their parent's care. The ACO nurse still visits monthly to try to prevent medication error and prevent duplicate therapy given that there are multiple prescribing physicians.*

Patient Engagement Capacity:

We believe that the ability for the patient to engage in their own care or in a therapeutic relationship with their care providers is the most important patient factor we observed. Engagement capacity can be affected by psychiatric disease, cognitive disorders, or overwhelming physical disease.

Patient engagement is a broad concept that builds on patient activation, a patient's skills, ability, knowledge, and willingness to manage their health. Engagement is associated with positive behaviors such as compliance with healthcare maintenance or maintaining a healthy diet and weight [8]. Engagement is strengthened as the result of treatment of significant depression, forming an alliance with supportive family members, and creating structured clear treatment and follow-up plans.

A person's engagement capacity can be influenced by their level of health literacy, educational level, their beliefs about the patient role, and/or a psychiatric illness including cognitive impairment. Engagement between a patient and the anchoring provider may be significantly challenged when the patient's disease is very complex and renders them physically unable to engage or often, as described in these narratives, when manifestations of psychiatric disease limit their capacity. Anchoring providers tend to know their patients well and often recognize the patients' limitations to engage. In response, they sustain and foster these relationships by engaging in a myriad of strategies. Some approach the patient cautiously, waiting for the right moment to engage the patient in a treatment conversation, some form alliances with family members, crafting strategies to help the patient manage their own care, while others use humor or other techniques to bolster the patient's capacity to participate in their care.

Our narratives revealed psychiatric illness as a frequent barrier to engagement. The following case study of MW, a 44-year-old man with multimorbid disease including depression and anxiety, illustrates the difficulty his provider and team encountered in monitoring his ongoing health status:

> *His next visit on 3/18/13 was arranged at the insistence of his wife. According to MW, he was still using his CPAP machine and his anxiety was under control. I asked if he had had follow-up with the sleep laboratory, He said "no". He continued to refuse recommended laboratory tests. I asked about blood sugars at home. He said he had stopped monitoring these as his time was "too valuable" and his partners were pressuring him to complete work. I was alarmed about his cavalier attitude about his medical care.*

Ms. X, a 14-year-old female with anorexia nervosa, was willing to engage with her primary care provider but not willing to engage with psychiatry due to perceived stigma. In this case, the primary care provider had a significant therapeutic alliance with the patient and parents and had successfully navigated anorexia treatment without relapse at 2-year follow-up.

> *I discussed the options of counseling and referral to a physiatrist for management of psychotropic medication. Nonetheless, the patient resisted seeing a psychiatrist because she didn't "want to be labeled" (thought of as "crazy"). I was disappointed but agreed instead to closely monitor her psychiatric status during frequent visits to medical appointments.*

This case was likely to succeed in part because the PCP was able to take advantage of this therapeutic alliance and use it to her advantage, and the subsequent advantage to the patient:

> *As an alternative to psychiatric referral I proposed treating X regularly with osteopathic manipulative treatment "for injuries and joint pain," recognizing the likely palliative (psychological) value of such a recommendation. I also told the patient's mother that regular visits could all me to follow X closely and intervene if there was more weight loss. It is worth noting here that in primary care medicine such "strategic" clinical moves are often necessary for engaging patients to follow an established treatment regimen and to stay away from counterproductive treatments.*

The ability to engage in self-care can be impacted by cognitive impairment as demonstrated in the case of Mr. B who suffered embolic strokes resulting in memory impairment, which resulted in his inability to manage his complex medication regimen. The physician recounts how she and her staff relied on his wife to help with his care, but she too suffered from diminished engagement capacity due to her own illness:

> *At first we attributed her lack of reliability in keeping appointments to her having to run the family business while caring for her seriously disabled husband, but later brain cancer was implicated. She was hospitalized for brain surgery an hour away from home, preventing her from caring for her cognitively impaired husband. In spite of homecare, and in her absence,*

he skipped several doses of furosemide triggering CHF and a potential hospitalization that I as the primary care physician was able to prevent because I was quite familiar with the patient's circumstances.

Lack of patient engagement affects providers and their teams as well as families/ caregivers, who heroically do everything in their power to assist the patient and when the patient cannot or will not engage often feel demoralized. The patient risks losing valuable advocates as demonstrated in the case of Roger, a 21-year T5 paraplegic with acute and chronic pain leading to physical dependence to opioids:

The patient's manipulations to obtain pain medications and his lack of compliance with treatment were discouraging to the medical staff who progressively became disaffected with a patient they originally championed. Family disillusionment and discord also played a significant role in hospital staff becoming disaffected with the patient. In addition, as the patient's failure to progress became intolerable to the parents their blame toward his caregivers including his physicians grew.

Social Support:

The concept of social support as applied to health care is complex, but simply put social support is associated with the perception that one is provided for and cared for. What generally follows are better self-management practices and improved health outcomes. Social support can be organized formally, such as from healthcare organizations, or informally, such as from family and friends [9, 10]. Studies have demonstrated four categories of social support: emotional, tangible, informational, and companionship [11]; social support can be either positive or negative.

Numerous studies highlight the importance of social support for improving patient treatment adherence, as well as having a positive effect on morbidity and mortality [12]. The provision of social support comes from family or significant others, and/or may manifest as "hands-on caregiving," encouragement and coaching to follow prescribed medical treatment plans and adopt healthy lifestyles, such as quitting smoking and exercising. It is important for the provider to be able to assess a patient's social support, especially when the patient has significant deficits in engagement capacity. Sadly, many complex cases involve patients who are isolated and have estranged relationships with family members.

Many of our narratives demonstrate the value of social support, where, without it, patients may have suffered tragic consequences as demonstrated by this case of a man with severe depression whose wife and provider formed a close therapeutic alliance allowing him to be successfully treated as an outpatient:

"It was there that he met his wife Maureen who would become his "rock", the source of stability in his life and his reason for living despite his deep pessimism". "He was unable to function without the assistance of his wife. Had it not been for her constant presence hospitalization would certainly have been necessary."

John was clearly at high risk for suicide and I recommended hospitalization. He was terrified of a psychiatric hospitalization since it would involve being separated from his wife, and pleaded with me to find an alternative. In response, his wife promised to supervise his day-to-day activities at home and monitor his medications. He agreed tentatively to initiate treatment with daily outpatient sessions combined with aggressive use of medications. I saw John daily, both individually and with his wife.

A therapeutic alliance with an "anchor" family member can contribute significantly to a positive outcome for the patient. Family, as social support, often has intimate knowledge of the patient and is a powerful partner to meet patient and provider goals:

The patient's mother identified concern about the patient's weight loss prior to the patient's first visit. The patient's mother followed the patient's care closely and formed an alliance with me supporting her daughter's care.

Family dynamics can often be complicated and may contribute to inhibiting a therapeutic relationship with the patient, and this may be especially apparent with pediatric patients. For example,

The family was in disarray. The support system I pictured within the family did not exist. Five months after their son's becoming paraplegic his parents were unsuccessfully struggling to cope with their own personal tragedy, not to mention its serious financial consequences.

Interestingly, the family dynamics in lives of sick or troubled children are often quite undependable. Their parents may have trouble coping themselves, may be overburdened by their child's illness, or may simply be opposed to professionals' advice about how to treat their child's illness or emotional dysfunction. In contrast to examples we have given of social support "shoring a patient up," parental overreaching can have a negative impact on a developing child as demonstrated by the following narrative of a 14-year-old male with seizure disorder and behavioral difficulties:

From this point, BB's parents, frightened for his health and safety began to monitor his every move. His father, in particular, knew every detail about his habits as if he alone could assure thathis already "damaged" child would love a life with any further harm, physically or emotional.

During this period BB was treated by a psychotherapist who repeatedly supported BB's growing desire to be free of his parents' well-intentioned but unremitting control. At this point virtually every attempt to set up an agenda for BB's progressive treatment was countermanded by his parents.

"Of note, his severely impoverished social life continued unchanged. It was difficult to motivate him to interact with peers. He repeatedly said the he "preferred to stay home after school and on week-ends and read books." He seemed to have little motivation to expend the effort or withstand the anxiety associated with making changes in his social and school related life, explaining that his parents were "so controlling: that it wasn't worth trying. Every move he made would be "criticized: new rules to "protect" him would be set."

Families/caregivers providing social support also find themselves in need of resources, leaving patients vulnerable, as evidenced by the following narratives. In these cases, the caregivers, formal and informal found themselves in need of support:

This patent's wife was distracted by the real-world work need to maintain the family business, which compromised her ability/willingness to care for him. This left him unsupervised which proved problematic when he could not manage his medications safely. During this period, his wife, the primary caretaker, developed a brain tumor further complicating her husband's management despite the addition of in-home care support.

In this example of an older man, frail and with complex illnesses, retired and divorced with minimal personal support, the informal caregiver, a neighbor, and paramedic also became ill and could no longer care for the patient, leaving only distant relatives to speak for him:

His background health and adjustment was one of marginal independence. He was watched over by a neighbor who also happened to be a paramedic and his granddaughter who lived on the East Coast and communicated frequently but did not have a local presence.

Patients and providers may have ideas or assumptions about social support that are incongruent with the patient and/or patient's circumstances:

Although she was largely estranged from her children she expected them to find roommates and help her with money for dental work. One daughter lives in a nearby town. Her son rarely spoke to her and lived about a two-hour drive away. Her youngest daughter and grandson lived in southern California about a one-day drive away and also would visit on holidays. Typically her depression would worsen around holidays and when her ex-husband would host the children for parties, cruises and other vacations including his new wife but excluding her.

He claimed that he preferred a socially isolated existence emphasizing "thinking" and had found a way to make his philosophical bent of mind a profession. In response, I said that while I appreciate his solace in solitude, choosing this mode of being might not work as well for him when depressed. At such times he might need to be more connected to others.

Conclusion

We have used interpretive narrative analysis to examine 16 complex case narratives written by PCPs and specialists who had cared for these patients in their practices. We identified patient, provider, and health system factors that we feel are particularly associated with patient engagement and outcome. The identified patient factors that were either barriers or facilitators for treatment were patient chaos, presence of social support, resource availability, and engagement/self-care capacity. System and provider factors identified were the provides' ability to create and maintain therapeutic and collaborative alliances and provider/team ability to discern and assess for these patient factors, including the presence of behavioral health issues.

We offer a conceptual model which shows the interaction and balance or imbalance between these factors, and how these factors may compensate for each other to keep the patient or case from becoming "complex" or move it further toward greater "complexity."

Our provider narratives are congruent with the literature in describing the challenges of managing complexity in primary care. A systematic review and synthesis of qualitative research on PCP perspectives on managing multimorbidity revealed [13] similar challenges: (1) a fragmented and disorganized healthcare system with multiple specialists and poorly coordinated care and communication leaving PCPs feeling excluded; (2) lack of adequate guidelines for managing multimorbidity; (3) providing patient-centered care may in fact lead to conflicts between specialists and

PCPs; and (4) shared decision making between provider and patient is difficult in the presence of many patient characteristics that are common in complex patients and cases, such as cognitive problems, lack of resources, poor social supports and low levels of patient engagement.

Health systems are often structured to manage one or two diseases at a time, but not the complexity of multimorbid health conditions. Complex patients require a long-term investment for providers and the health system, as the diseases themselves, resources, social support, and patient engagement wax and wane over time. Additional constraints are many and for example include a deficiency of evidence-based treatment recommendations for complex health conditions, reimbursement policies that lead to shortened office visits, and the lack of investment in team care models. Patients with significant complex disease are usually difficult to manage and require major investments of a provider's time, creativity, compassion, and persistence. Highly skilled practitioners are required to assess, plan, and manage these patient and health system factors.

References

1. Kathol RG, Perez R, Cohen. The integrated case management manual. Assisting complex patients regain physical and mental health. New York: Springer Publishing Company, LLC; 2010.
2. Stifel FC, deJonge P, Huyse FJ, Guex P, Slaets JP, Lyons JS, et al. "INTERMED": a method to assess health service needs. II. Results on its validity and clinical use. Gen Hosp Psychiatry. 1999;21(1):49–56.
3. Peek CJ, Baird M, Coleman E. An orientation to complexity assessment and draft of the "Minnesota Complexity Assessment Method". University of Minnesota, Working draft, 2009.
4. Loeb DF, Binswanger IA, Candrian C, Bayliss EA. Primary care physician insights into a typology of the complex patient in primary care. Ann Fam Med. 2015;13(5):451–5.
5. Denzin NK, Lincoln YS. The sage handbook of qualitative research. Thousand Oaks: Sage Publications; 2005.
6. Benner P. The tradition and skill of interpretive phenomenology in studying health, illness, and caring practices. In: Benner P, editor. Interpretive phenomenology: embodiment, caring and ethics in health and illness. Thousand Oaks: Sage; 1994. p. 99–128.
7. Bayliss EA, Steiner JF, Fernald DH, Crane LA, Main DS. Descriptions of barriers to self-care by persons with comorbid chronic diseases. Ann Fam Med. 2003;1(1):15–21.
8. James J, Hibbard J, Agres T, Lott R, Dentzer S. Health policy brief: patient engagement. Health Aff. 2013;33(6):1–6.
9. van Dam HA, van der Horst FG, Knoops L, Ryckman RM, Crebolder HFJM, van den Borne BHW. Social support in diabetes: a systematic review of controlled intervention studies. Patient Educ Couns. 2005;59:1–12.
10. Bardach SH, Tarasenko YN, Schoenberg NE. Therold of social support in multiple morbidity: self-management amoung rural residents. J Health Care Poor Underserved. 2011;22(3):756–71.
11. Ford ME, Tilley BC, McDonald PE. Social support among African American adults with diabetes, part 1: theoretical framework. J Natl Med Assoc. 1998;90(6):361–5.
12. Berkman LF, Leo-Summers L, Horwitz RI. Emotional support and survival after myocardial infarction: a prospective population based study of the elderly. Ann Intern Med. 1992;117:1003.
13. Sinnott C, Mc Hugh S, Browne J, Bradley C. GPs' perspectives on the management of patients with multimorbidity: systematic review and synthesis of qualitative research. BMJ Open. 2013;3:e003610. https://doi.org/10.1136/bmjopen-2013-003610.

Chapter 25
Reflections and Conclusions

Steven A. Frankel and James A. Bourgeois

In effect, this is an "adventure book." True, it is technical, offering the distillate of years of experience and accumulated wisdom from roughly 20 medical experts, mainly physicians. The terrain is that of multiple medical specializations, including the entities constituting primary care, family medicine, and internal medicine. Each is a delimited world enveloping a defined group of physicians. For example, the environment of pediatrics is vastly different from that of pain medicine, even when there is some overlap. The common factor for both, however, is, of course, *people* – the sick and otherwise compromised patients who we treat. The other main commonality is the importance we as treaters have to our patients, not so different from the leader of a climbing expedition who is responsible for each climber. In that case, your welfare and perhaps your life is in the leader's hands. If you have ever been seriously ill or hospitalized and fully dependent on medical providers, you know what we mean. Drs. Graf and Intinarelli (Chap. 24) make this point clearly when they emphasize the central importance of the "therapeutic relationship" to medical outcome, its palliative and curative value having been repeatedly confirmed in the medical literature. Of interest is our observation that the ideal location for treating complex cases is likely to be in the community, since it is there that a treatment relationship is most likely to be developed and sustained [1–3].

S.A. Frankel, MD (✉)
Department of Psychiatry, University of California, School of Medicine, San Francisco, CA, USA
e-mail: saf@stevenfrankelmd.com

J.A. Bourgeois
Department of Psychiatry, Baylor Scott & White Health, Central Texas Division, Temple, TX, USA

Department of Psychiatry, Texas A and M University Health Sciences Center, College of Medicine, Temple, TX, USA

Department of Psychiatry, University of California San Francisco, School of Medicine, San Francisco, CA, USA
e-mail: James.Bourgeois@BSWHealth.org

© Springer International Publishing AG, part of Springer Nature 2018
S.A. Frankel, J.A. Bourgeois (eds.), *Integrated Care for Complex Patients*,
https://doi.org/10.1007/978-3-319-61214-0_25

We hope you have joined with our pediatricians, internists, nurses, and sleep specialists, among others, as they have taken you through the challenges and repeatedly tense moments of their clinical work. If asked to summarize what you have read as it applies to your own work how would you do that? We will try our hand at this, but we are fully aware of the crucial pieces we will leave out. These are mainly the subjective "filler" contributions that pervade clinical work: the wisdom, commitment, integrity, and, yes, impatience that those who chose to work with patients, especially complex patients and complex cases, invariably bring to their practices.

Technical contributions include choosing to work with and understand complex patients and cases with multiple medical, and particularly medical-psychiatric, comorbidities. Notice that there are no cases in our collection of narratives that are without psychiatric comorbidity. This is striking, in a way, since psychiatric comorbidity, as well as social dysfunction, has traditionally been deemphasized in general medicine. The biological basis of medicine is of course always there and evolving. Technology, including laboratory studies and diagnostic imaging, is hard to keep up with. However, psychiatric, social, and sociological factors are often intertwined with systemic medical considerations, and the pathogenic effect of each is often hard to separate.

As our case narratives illustrate, nothing is as complex as the person we treat and his or her associated personal and interpersonal environment. The contributing factors include the "imponderables" in medical practice, the elusive factors that slow or prevent a patient's healing or promote healing at an unexpected rate. Further complicating this part of the treatment process is its duration, with biological and environmental factors shifting during treatment. In effect, the "terrain" and "weather" are always changing and "climbing conditions" are as well. Dr. Clark-Sayles' patient impeded her own treatment by being self-willed and refusing to honor her treating physician's recommendations; Dr. Palistrant's anorexia nervosa patient was not forthcoming and thereby obscured her diagnosis and treatment requirements. The parents in Dr. Mendius' case involving two brothers refused to consider that the basic problem afflicting their sons could be psychiatric. Dr. Lau watched with frustration as his patient became indigent, and both he and the patient realized that needed medical care was out of reach within his public health system. In contrast, for Dr. Gilbert's depressed man, the involvement of his wife made it possible for him to recover from severe depression and to do so without hospitalization.

We could capture the complexity of our cases by focusing on psychiatric-systemic medical comorbidity, as well as social and health systems factors [4]. But, even then we are unlikely to find a fully coherent framework from which to describe and make predictions for these complicated cases, especially if we want to include the associated microscopic influences and shifting levels of complexity. And yet, complex clinical cases are a major challenge within our health-care system. Public clinics and private offices are virtually flooded with these patients. Drs. Graf and Intinarelli (Chap. 24) do an exemplary job of incorporating and naming these myriad of complexity factors. In their chapter, they make it clear that prioritizing these contributions can only be done on a clinical basis, taking into consideration the patient's interaction with a treating physician.

Our case narratives illustrate these complexities. They are organized by the medical specialty. Each chapter begins with an extended case narrative, followed by physician reflections. A list of complexity factors and their relative contribution to the challenge of managing that case follows. Factors included in that list are (1) biological (including genetic); (2) psychiatric/psychological; (3) social stressors (including the contribution of family and the lack of needed support personnel); (4) care delivery, including access to care; and (5) fundamental factors supporting or obstructing treatment, in particular the quality and continuity of the physician-patient relationship.

Shifting from clinical considerations to treatment requirements, we make recommendations in the first six chapters of this book for managing complex cases both in community and major medical center settings. The required personnel, including case managers, and clinical screening tools for working up and triaging these cases are described. Each clinical case, including its financial requirements, can be a challenge for treating clinicians. The "big picture" goal always includes the "triple aim" of improved care for individuals and populations, as well as cost savings [5].

Over the last 20 years, increasing numbers of physicians have pursued combined postgraduate residencies in both psychiatry and primary care specialties (primarily family medicine or internal medicine) and psychiatry. Consistent with the adoption of a population health focus emphasizing utilization patterns, the motivation for this development is likely a greater appreciation of the existence and abundance of "complex patients" as explicated in this book. Physicians dually skilled in primary care and psychiatry may be the most appropriate physicians for the ongoing care of these complex patients and the associated complex cases.

As illustrated by the case narratives in this book, many patients are experienced as complex because of the baseline existence of comorbidity consisting of chronic systemic and psychiatric illness. Physicians skilled both in primary care specialties and in psychiatry are well prepared to take full responsibility at the interfaces encountered when managing clinical complexity. Ironically, systems of care have sometimes struggled with the best way to deploy these dually trained physicians. Some of the created but circumscribed roles for them have included consultation-liaison psychiatry, and psychiatric and primary care of the chronically mentally ill. However, the prospect of using dually trained physicians more specifically as what might be called "clinical complexity specialists" may be especially attractive and timely, since it both optimizes the care of complex patients and could provide a meaningful and rewarding career path for broadly trained physicians.

A source of complexity not mentioned so far in this chapter is the confusing array of treatment possibilities available in the community. In Chap. 5, we catalog types of community-based health-care providers and methods of care delivery. The abundance of possibilities makes the health-care scene more ambiguous than might be anticipated. It reduces the likelihood of patients getting the same level and quality of health care for the same type of problem from different sources. This area of complexity is represented in our case narratives. A prominent example is Dr. Lau's patient encountering institutional limitations, as he required transfer from one facility to another. In other situations, the differences between providers and facilities are likely to be more subtle but no less relevant for treatment outcome.

In Chap. 6 we search for solutions to the care delivery challenges that plague the health-care system. To that end, we have proposed that "clinical/medical complexity" be accorded a place as a formal *specialization* within medicine or as a *medical specialty* itself [6]. Achieving this end will be demanding as a precise set of definitions and their associated limits are identified. It will be necessary to make sure that activities subsumed within the category "clinical/medical complexity" do not unreasonably overlap those of other specialty areas within medicine. In keeping with this recommendation, we also propose that *specific referral and treatment centers* be created for complex clinical cases. Detailed proposals for creating this new medical specialization/specialty and for the structure and administration of "complexity centers" will be developed in our future publications.

Our hope is that this book has served to bring order to the not-so-orderly subject of clinical/medical complexity, assisting both clinicians and health-care administrators to understand and deal with complex clinical situations. We hope that our collaborative discussion group, The Center for Collaborative Medicine, Psychiatry, and Psychology, can serve as a model to other groups interested in sharing interests and information in medicine. Aiding our endeavor has been the work of others who have committed themselves to understand clinical complexity, namely, the Intermed consortium in Europe and Roger Kathol, MD in the USA. Anyone who has undertaken a difficult climbing expedition will tell you that the array of factors complicating their effort is unending, and that the outcome is far from predictable. Having reliable help along the way is imperative. Such is the challenge of clinical medicine devoted to complex cases and their treatments, but the excitement of it as well.

References

1. Frankel R. Relationship-centered care and the patient-physician relationship. J Gen Intern Med. 2004;19(11):1163–5.
2. Gittell JH. High performance healthcare: using the power of relationships to achieve quality, efficiency and resilience. New York: McGraw-Hill; 2009.
3. Norcross JC, editor. Psychotherapy relationships that work: therapist contributions and responsiveness to patients needs. New York: Oxford University Press; 2002.
4. Kathol R, Denhel P, Knutson K. Physician's Guide to understanding and working with integrated case managers. New York: Springer; 2016.
5. Institute for Healthcare Improvement. IHI Triple Aim Initiative. Website: http://www.ihi.org/Engage/Initiatives/TripleAim/Pages/default.aspx. 2017.
6. Holland, J. Hidden Order: How adaptation builds complexity. Illustrated. Addison-Wesley Publishing Company; 1995.

Index

© Springer International Publishing AG, part of Springer Nature 2018
S.A. Frankel, J.A. Bourgeois (eds.), *Integrated Care for Complex Patients*,
https://doi.org/10.1007/978-3-319-61214-0